EASY WAY TO STOP SMOKING

"It is a remarkable fact that Allen Carr, on his own admission a non-professional in behaviour modification, should have succeeded where countless psychologists and psychiatrists holding post-graduate qualifications have failed, in formulating a *SIMPLE* and *EFFECTIVE* way to stop smoking." *Dr William Green MB; Chb; FRANZCP; MRCPsych; DPM. Head of the Psychiatric Department, Matilda Hospital, Hong Kong.*

"I was really impressed by the method. In spite of Allen Carr's success and fame, there were no gimmicks and the professional approach was something a GP could really respect. I would be happy to give a medical endorsement of the method to anyone."*Dr P. M. Bray, MB, Chb, MRCGP, Barnet General Hospital, UK*

"I have observed the Allen Carr method, "The Easy Way To Stop Smoking", at first hand on several occasions. I have found it to be very successful. I wholeheartedly support it as an effective way to quit smoking."
Dr Anil Visram BSc. MBBch. FRCA. Consultant, The Royal Hospitals Trust, Royal London Hospital, UK.

"I was exhilarated by a new sense of freedom."
The Independent

"An intelligent and original method"
Evening Standard

ABOUT THE AUTHOR

For a third of a century Allen Carr chain-smoked 60 to 100 cigarettes a day. He was a successful accountant, but his addiction was driving him to despair. In 1983, after countless failed attempts to quit, by using will-power and other methods, he finally discovered what the world had been waiting for – the *Easy Way to Stop Smoking*. Since leaving accountancy to help cure the world's smokers, he has built up a global reputation as a result of his phenomenal method. Smokers used to have to fly from all over the world to attend his clinic in London; now his network of clinics spans the globe. *Allen Carr's Easy Way to Stop Smoking* is an international bestseller and has been published in over twenty different languages. His second book, *The Only Way to Stop Smoking Permanently*, and video, audio and CD-ROM versions of his method are also available. In his third publication, *Allen Carr's Easyweigh to Lose Weight*, he applies the same simple logic to weight-loss, so that it becomes easy and enjoyable, as those attending his clinics have discovered. His other titles are *How to Stop Your Child Smoking*, *The Easy Way To Enjoy Flying*, *The Easy Way To Control Alcohol*, and *The Easy Way for Women to Stop Smoking*, as well as a range of inspirational books, including *No More Worrying*, *No More Hangovers* and *No More Diets*.

Allen Carr was invited to speak at the 10th World Conference on Tobacco & Health held in Beijing in 1998, an honour that the most eminent physician would be proud of. His method and reputation could receive no higher commendation. He is now widely accepted as the world's leading expert on how to help smokers to quit.

A full list of Allen Carr clinics appears at the back of this book. Should you require any assistance, do not hesitate to contact your nearest therapist. Weight-control sessions are now offered at selected clinics. A full corporate service is also available, enabling companies to implement no-smoking policies simply and effectively. All correspondence and enquiries about Allen Carr's books, videos, audio tapes and CD-ROMs should be addressed to the nearest clinic.

ALLEN CARR
EASY WAY TO
STOP
SMOKING

ARCTURUS

ARCTURUS

This edition published in 2011 by Arcturus Publishing Limited
26/27 Bickels Yard, 151–153 Bermondsey Street,
London SE1 3HA

ISBN: 978-1-905555-29-1
AD000032EN

Printed in China

To Robin Hayley

CONTENTS

PREFACE

Just suppose there were a magic method of stopping smoking which enables any smoker, including you, to quit:

- IMMEDIATELY!
- PERMANENTLY!
- WITHOUT SUFFERING WITHDRAWAL SYMPTOMS!
- WITHOUT PUTTING ON WEIGHT!
- WITHOUT USING SHOCK TACTICS, PILLS, PATCHES OR OTHER GIMMICKS!

Let's further suppose that:

- THERE IS NO INITIAL FEELING OF DEPRIVATION OR MISERY!
- YOU IMMEDIATELY ENJOY SOCIAL OCCASIONS MORE!
- YOU FEEL MORE CONFIDENT AND BETTER EQUIPPED TO HANDLE STRESS!
- YOU ARE BETTER ABLE TO CONCENTRATE!
- YOU DON'T SPEND THE REST OF YOUR LIFE HAVING TO RESIST THE OCCASIONAL TEMPTATION TO LIGHT A CIGARETTE – AND
- YOU NOT ONLY FIND IT EASY TO QUIT, BUT CAN ACTUALLY ENJOY THE PROCESS FROM THE MOMENT YOU EXTINGUISH THAT LAST CIGARETTE!

If there were such a magical method, would you use it? You'd be pretty stupid not to. But, of course, you don't believe in magic. Neither do I. Nevertheless, the method I describe above certainly does exist. I call it Easyway. In fact, it isn't magic, it just seems that way. It certainly seemed that way to me when I first discovered it and I know that many of the millions of ex-smokers who have successfully quit with the help of Easyway also view it in that light.

No doubt you still find my claims difficult to believe. Don't worry, I would regard you as somewhat naive if you just accepted them without proof. On the other hand, don't make the mistake of dismissing them because you believe they are grossly exaggerated. In all probability you are only reading this book because of the recommendation of an ex-smoker who attended an Easyway clinic or read this book.

It matters not whether you received the recommendation directly or through someone who loves you and is desperately worried that, unless you quit, you won't be there to go on loving.

Does this mean that you will also need to visit an Easyway clinic? No. There is only one Easyway method. How does it work? That is not easy to describe briefly. Smokers arrive at our clinics in different states of panic, convinced that they won't succeed and believing that even if by some miracle they do manage to quit, they will first have to endure an indeterminable period of abject misery, that social occasions will never be quite so enjoyable, that they will be less able to concentrate and cope with stress and that, although they might never smoke again, they will never be completely free and that for the rest of their lives they will have occasional yearnings to smoke a cigarette and will have to resist the temptation.

Eighty percent of those smokers leave the clinic a few hours later already happy non-smokers. How do we achieve that miracle? You need to book an appointment at an Easyway clinic to find out. However, what I can say is that most smokers expect us to achieve that objective by telling them of the terrible health risks that they run, that smoking is a dirty, disgusting habit, that it costs them a fortune and how stupid they are not to quit. No, we do not patronize them by telling them what they already know. These are problems of being a smoker. They are not problems of quitting. Smokers do not smoke for the reasons why they shouldn't smoke. In order to quit it is necessary to remove the reasons why we do smoke. Easyway addresses this problem. It removes the desire to smoke. Once the desire to smoke has been removed, the ex-smoker doesn't need to use will-power.

The Easyway method exists in the form of clinics, books, videos, audio tapes, CD-ROM and Internet courses. In each case the method is the same but simply uses different vehicles to communicate it. Which vehicle should you use? It's a question of personal choice. Some people prefer reading books, others prefer watching videos. In this pack you have the method in book form, backed up by two CDs.

The clinics enjoy such a high success rate that we are able to give a money-back guarantee. The drawback of other products is that if you fail to understand or disagree with a particular point, you cannot raise it with the therapist, and if you miss an important point the product has no way of correcting the situation. At the clinics you have the benefit of an experienced therapist. Our therapists are all ex-smokers who quit with the benefit of Easyway. They are carefully selected and meticulously trained to be sympathetic to your needs. You are able to question points that you either do not understand or agree with. On the other hand if you unknowingly misunderstand an important point the therapist will invariably be aware of it and correct the situation.

Another main advantage of the clinic is that you are in congenial surroundings with nothing to distract you from the main objective. Although the atmosphere on arrival can resemble that of the dentist's waiting room, it soon transforms into that of a happy reunion of old friends as you identify and relate to the other members of the group. However, the main advantage of the clinic is that your problem becomes our responsibility. The fee varies according to location and, if you are one of the 20 percent who require more than one visit, you can attend any number of follow-ups without further charge. Our motto is similar to that of the Royal Canadian Mounted Police – 'we never give up on our man (or woman)'. If you decide that you no longer wish to quit, your fee will be refunded in full. On the basis of the money-back guarantee, the world-wide success rate at our clinics averages over 90 percent.

Do not let any of the above distract you from the value of this pack. It is a complete course in itself, and thousands of smokers have quit easily simply by reading the book alone. If you are in doubt, why not telephone your nearest clinic for further guidance. (A list of clinics is provided at the back of the book.)

1

HOW CAN A BOOK HELP YOU TO QUIT?

If you have read other books that purport to help you to quit, you will already believe that they can't. Perhaps you are expecting me to tell you how stupid you are for being a smoker and what a weak-willed, spineless jellyfish you are because so far you've failed to quit. If so, I assure you, you could not be more wrong. I've no doubt that you'll be expecting me to shock you with horror stories about the terrible damage you are doing to your lungs, of the thousands of pounds that will literally go up in smoke and the lifetime of lethargy, wheezing, coughing, slavery, filth and self-disgust. Again I must disappoint you.

So am I going to appeal to you to think how worried your family and friends are because you smoke and ask you to use a little will-power and discipline? After all, millions of adult smokers have successfully quit in recent years, so why can't you? No, that isn't my technique either. If you have read other books on quitting smoking you will no doubt be expecting to absorb pages and pages of charts and statistics informing you of such things as how many years you will lose from your life if you smoke X number of cigarettes per day. You will be pleased to learn that there are no charts in this book.

So what else is there to know and why do I waste your time and mine by telling you what you might or might not be expecting me to say? Why don't I just come right out and tell you just how Easyway works? Because we are in a chicken and egg situation. When I first discovered the 'magic' button that released me immediately and permanently from the nicotine trap, I believed that I could cure any smoker within five minutes. I knew that it was possible to help all smokers to find it easy to quit. What I didn't realize was how difficult it is to convince some smokers that they too can find it easy to quit. There are two main obstacles. The first is:

FEAR

No matter how calm they might appear on the surface, smokers arrive at our clinics in various stages of panic. They have several basic fears:
• Will I be a failure? And even if I do succeed, will I have to go through an indeterminate period of misery and deprivation?

• Will I ever enjoy a meal or social occasion again?
• Will I be able to answer the telephone or cope with stress?
• Will life ever be quite the same again?
• Will I ever be completely free?

A few hours later, over 90 percent of them leave already happy non-smokers, immediately able to enjoy social occasions more and better equipped to cope with stress.

If Easyway will work for any smoker, why do some smokers fail? There are several reasons. A major one is fear. As a smoker you will certainly suffer from some, and probably all, of the fears I have just mentioned. It is these fears that make us desperately search for any flimsy excuse to postpone what we think of as the evil day we have to quit smoking and make us block our minds to the stupidity of being a smoker.

Fear impedes good understanding and this is where the chicken and egg situation arises. If there were a magic button that you could press so that you could wake up tomorrow morning already a happy non-smoker, as if you had never been a smoker, enjoying social occasions more, feeling better equipped to handle stress, never having the slightest temptation to smoke a cigarette or feeling that there was a void in your life without smoking and looking at other smokers, not with envy, but with genuine pity as you would for someone that was forced to inject heroin into their veins, would you press that button?

If you have hesitated to arrive at your answer, the only plausible reason is fear, the belief that the magic button won't work:

EASYWAY IS THAT MAGIC BUTTON!

2

THE PRISONER

Imagine a doctor saying to a prisoner:

"It's damp in here and you're suffering from pneumonia. You are clearly undernourished and your family is very worried about you. Now why don't you be a sensible fellow and go home?"

The doctor giving that advice would not only be regarded as patronizing but incredibly stupid. He is simply telling the prisoner what he already knows. What the prisoner really needs is not someone telling him how stupid he is, but someone who will give him the key to the prison.

Smokers are in exactly the same position. You might argue that they are not. The prisoner has no choice but the smoker has. No one forces him to smoke and if he decides that he no longer wants to, who can prevent him from stopping? That sounds very logical, but you cannot disregard the fact that several times in my life I made the decision that I never wanted to smoke again, but I didn't succeed.

You could argue that the only reason that I didn't succeed was because, having attempted to quit, it eventually dawned on me that a smoker's life was more enjoyable than that of a non-smoker. If that were true, I'd still be a smoker. The true reason that I didn't succeed was that I didn't know how to escape from that prison.

If smokers were able to quit just like that, you would have no need to read this book and doctors would have no need to tell smokers what they already know. Let's accept the simple fact that, although there are no visible iron bars, if a smoker wants to quit but cannot, he is effectively imprisoned whether he likes it or not.

Let's also accept that your reasons for wanting to leave a prison, although they give you the desire to escape, don't necessarily help you to do so. Suppose you were given an hour to solve a complicated problem. If you were then told that your very life depended on arriving at the correct solution, do you think that you would be more likely to solve it, or do you think that panic would ensure that you didn't solve it?

Other so-called experts and smokers themselves find it difficult to accept that their reasons for stopping, no matter how powerful those reasons might be, not only don't help them to quit, but actually make it harder, and the more powerful they are, the harder they make it.

This might appear illogical to you but just think: does dieting make food appear to be less precious or ten times more so?

Get it clearly into your mind: we don't smoke for the reasons that we shouldn't smoke. If you want to be a non-smoker, you need to remove the reasons that make you want to smoke.

Surely the more powerful your reasons for stopping the easier it should be to quit? There are several reasons why this is not so:

- It creates a feeling of sacrifice and deprivation. We are being forced to give up our pleasure or crutch.
- The more powerful your reasons are for stopping, the more your subconscious brain will deduce: "I must either get some tremendous pleasure or crutch from smoking, or the hold it has over me must be all powerful, otherwise I wouldn't still be smoking and neither would all these other idiots."
- One of the occasions that smokers reach for a cigarette is during times of stress. If you tell a smoker it's killing them, this creates stress and makes the need for a cigarette even greater. This is why smokers block their minds to health warnings and why some tobacco companies actually use shock tactics to sell cigarettes.

But the most important reason is that it creates a bind: we always concentrate on the reasons why we shouldn't smoke. Easyway tackles the real problem: it removes the desire to smoke. You might still argue that if you tell a smoker that smoking causes lung cancer this will remove the desire to smoke.

In fact it doesn't. It might well enable that smoker to resist the temptation to smoke either in the short term or permanently, but it will no more remove the desire to smoke than you'll remove the hunger of a starving man by telling him that his food is poisoned.

Does this mean that smokers can never lose the desire to smoke? No; eating is natural, essential for survival and a genuine pleasure that can be enjoyed throughout our lives. Smoking is unnatural, destructive, unpleasant and a bane throughout our lives.

I'm not going to ask you to trust me or to rely on faith. I've referred to Easyway as that 'magic' button. Strictly this is not so. Although thousands of smokers including myself found the effects of Easyway magical, in fact there was no magic involved, it just seemed that way. On the contrary, it is based on pure reason and logic. A conjurer can perform a clever illusion that appears to be magical. However, once the illusion has been explained, we realize that there is no magic.

The nicotine trap is the most ingenious, subtle and sinister illusion that nature and mankind have ever combined to create. Abraham Lincoln said:

"You can fool all of the people some of the time and some of the people all of the time, but you can't fool all of the people all of the time."

For generations Abraham was wrong, because that is exactly what the tobacco industry had done: fooled all the people all of the time! But Abraham was right and I'm privileged to be the vehicle that proved him so. I was the first to explode the illusion of the nicotine trap. I would like to claim that I did so because of my incredible insight and intelligence. However, to be honest, it was really due to the particular circumstances of my life. A plant might send millions of seeds into the atmosphere. Perhaps only one seed will be fortunate enough to land in a spot where it can survive and reproduce.

As far as understanding the mysteries of the smoking illusion is concerned, I regard myself as that seed. However, I do credit myself for appreciating my good luck and having the courage to devote the remainder of my life to helping others to escape from nicotine addiction.

As I have said, fear impedes success. I've also said that I'm not going to ask you to trust me or to rely on faith. I promise that I will explain everything to you. But we need to break this chicken and egg situation. I can show you how to find it easy to quit, but I need your help. I need you to start off in the right frame of mind. There is no need to be frightened. Non-smokers don't get that panic feeling that smokers get when they run out of cigarettes late at night, and one of the great advantages of being free is to be rid of that fear.

Get into your mind that there is no need to feel frightened or miserable. Nothing bad is happening. On the contrary, something marvellous is happening. The only reason that you are reading this book is because you want to quit smoking. I'm going to show you the easy way to do it.

Perhaps you are still worried that I'm trying to bluff you or that my method won't work for you. Just think. For most of my life I was just one small rather insignificant human being. I don't have the vast resources of the established medical profession or the nicotine replacement conglomerates. You won't find me advertising my method. I have become famous for one reason and one reason alone:

MY METHOD WORKS AND IT WILL WORK FOR ANY SMOKER, INCLUDING YOU!

All you have to do to make it work is to follow the simple instructions that I give you. Remove any feelings of:

"Oh God! I've got to give up my crutch, my pleasure!"

Get it into your mind – there is nothing bad happening. The main reason that I started this book by telling you of all the things that I wasn't going to say was to make you realize that there is no need to feel miserable or depressed. There is no need to be afraid. I have only good news for you. You are about to achieve something that every smoker on this planet would love to achieve:

TO BE FREE!

Your second instruction right now is to:

START OFF WITH A FEELING OF ELATION

In case you missed the first instruction, and because it is the most important, I will repeat it. Your first instruction is:

TO FOLLOW ALL INSTRUCTIONS TO THE LETTER

I'm now going to ask you to do something that you might think is illogical. Bearing in mind that the sole object of this book is to help you to quit smoking, you might find that at various stages you have the inclination to quit immediately. I would ask you to resist any such temptation. At the end of the book I will explain the ritual of your final cigarette. It is imperative that you neither attempt to quit nor to cut down prior to that ritual.

THAT IS YOUR THIRD INSTRUCTION

This is the only instruction that can be broken, but only if you have already extinguished your final cigarette before you started reading this book, in which case it is essential that you finish the book as soon as possible. The instructions are listed at the back of the book for easy reference.

In the opening chapter I said that there were two main obstacles to success. The first was fear. The second is:

THE CLOSED MIND

3

THE CLOSED MIND

Although fear is the main reason that closes a smoker's mind, it is the closed mind itself which causes the failure. Are you a trusting person? Do you tend to believe what people tell you, to give them the benefit of the doubt? If so, for the purposes of this book, I need you to be the biggest sceptic on the planet. Can you imagine the problems Columbus must have had when he tried to convince people that the world was round?

"Round! How can it be round?"

"I assure you it is. The Australians are actually standing upside down."

"Nonsense, I've been to Australia. I wasn't upside down. In any case, why don't they fall off?"

"Because of gravity."

"What's gravity? Can you show me some?"

"Well, you can't actually see it, but it must be there. Otherwise Australians would fall off and so would we."

"Surely a more simple explanation is the world is flat!"

Even in this so-called enlightened age, society's general knowledge and understanding about smoking is equivalent to believing that the world is flat. My task isn't quite so difficult as Columbus's, although sometimes I wonder. I need you to be sceptical, not only of me, but of your own opinions about smoking and about what society has taught you about smoking. I need you to not only believe what I'm saying to you, but to understand what I'm saying and know that it is the truth, so that when you experience the joys of being free from nicotine addiction, nothing and no one can ever again delude you into believing that you need to smoke. Your fourth instruction is:

KEEP AN OPEN MIND

How can this book help you to quit smoking? A book is a means of communicating information. It can help you to achieve anything, whether it be for evil: like creating a bomb, or for good: like helping smokers to escape from the nicotine trap. But what information can Allen Carr give me that will help me to quit? I already know that it's not improving my health or helping my pocket. I know it's a filthy, disgusting habit. I also know that it's almost impossible to quit. So you think you know all you need to know about smoking? Let's put it to the test. Let's find out:

WHAT DO YOU REALLY KNOW ABOUT SMOKING?

4

WHAT DO YOU REALLY KNOW ABOUT SMOKING?

Answer a simple 'yes' or 'no' to the following questions. You might find it difficult to do that with certain of them.

In those cases, answer 'yes' or 'no' according to what you think the majority of people would answer.

1. Do people smoke because they choose to?
2. Do smokers enjoy smoking?
3. Do some cigarettes, for example the one after a meal, taste better than others?
4. Do some youngsters become smokers because:
   a. They think it's cool to smoke? and/or
   b. Because it makes them feel grown up? and/or
   c. Because they think smoking will give them confidence?
5. Do some smokers enjoy the taste of cigarettes?
6. Is smoking a habit?
7. Are heavy smokers more hooked than casual smokers?
8. Are smokers that have been smoking for years more hooked than youngsters who have just started?
9. Does smoking help to relieve boredom?
10. Does smoking aid concentration?
11. Does smoking help relaxation?
12. Does smoking help to relieve stress?
13. Does smoking help the nerves?
14. Are smokers stupid?
15. Does it take will-power to quit?
16. Do some people have addictive personalities?
17. Does smoking help to reduce weight?
18. Does it help to use nicotine replacement therapy (NRT); i.e. gum, patches or sprays containing nicotine?
19. Is it necessary to suffer from withdrawal symptoms when quitting?
20. Is it difficult to quit?

Since question 4 contains 3 separate questions, there are in fact 22 questions in all. The correct answer to every question is: NO.

If you read down the list again, I will forgive you for questioning my credibility. If I further tell you that not only do smokers not enjoy smoking, but that not a single smoker past or present has ever enjoyed smoking a single cigarette, you might not only question my credibility but my very sanity.

If you are tempted to despatch this book into the nearest dustbin, I would beg you to first hear me out. No matter how difficult you might find it to accept some of the statements that I make at this stage, I will prove to you that everything that I tell you is true.

Some of the illusions about smoking that smokers and society generally accept as fact can be dispelled quickly. Boredom and concentration are complete opposites. So are relaxing and stressful situations. Now, if I were to attempt to sell you a magic pill that would cure all evils and have the complete opposite effect to the same pill taken an hour earlier, you would have me locked up as a charlatan. Yet that is what smokers and society generally claim that smoking will do.

At this stage I must give you two warnings. At various stages you might feel tempted either to cut down on your smoking or even to quit completely before you have finished the book. Both could cause your failure. Remember Easyway will enable any smoker to actually find it enjoyable to quit, provided you follow all the instructions. Prior to the ritual of the last cigarette, if you have the slightest urge to smoke don't try to resist it, light up. You don't have to chain-smoke but if that is what you find yourself doing, don't worry about it.

There are two important reasons for continuing to smoke at this stage. Some people believe that one of them is to make you smoke more so that your lungs become so congested that smoking would cease to be a pleasure. It's called 'aversion' therapy. If it worked, I would use it, but aversion therapy will only work for as long as it takes your lungs to recover, a few days at the most.

One of the reasons that I need you to smoke at this stage is that we need to dispel the illusions. I've claimed that not a single smoker past or present has ever enjoyed smoking a single cigarette. That sounds an outrageous statement to make and there's no way I could possibly persuade you that it is true. I need you to prove it to yourself.

Between now and the ritual of your final cigarette I want you to become more aware of your smoking when you are actually smoking the cigarettes, particularly the so-called special ones, like the one after a meal. Ask yourself what it is that you are actually enjoying. Also observe other smokers, notice that once they have lit up, they don't appear to be aware that they are smoking. It seems to be automatic. Also observe how many of your own cigarettes were smoked subconsciously.

Let's start the process right now. Unless you are already smoking one, I want you to light a cigarette now. I want you to inhale as deeply as you can six times in succession. I want you to concentrate on the process and ask yourself where the pleasure is. At our clinics we ask a smoker who claims that they enjoy smoking to do this: the conversation usually goes something like this:

S: "No, I've just put one out. I don't want another one now."
Me: "Indulge yourself. If you really enjoy them, enjoy another."

By this time the other smokers in the group have sensed what is going to happen and have big grins on their faces. After the first puff the victim tries to change the conversation:

S: "I'm not particularly enjoying this one, it's really the one after a meal that I enjoy."
Me: "Why should the same cigarette out of the same packet taste different after a meal?"
S: "I don't know."
Me: "Tell me, if after a meal you can't smoke your particular brand of cigarettes and can only obtain a brand that you find distasteful, do you smoke it?"
S: "Of course I do."
Me: "Exactly. Smokers would rather smoke old rope than nothing! But you've only taken one puff, now please take the other five and sell it to me, tell me what marvellous experience you are having that I'm missing?"

Perhaps I've given the impression that we try to humiliate our clients at the clinics. I assure you this is not so. In the early days my wife acted as receptionist at the clinic. Joyce was one of those lucky people who as youngsters find their first cigarette so repulsive they are not tempted to light another. However, she was able to sense the panic feeling the smokers had when they first arrived, yet during the sessions she could hear frequent bursts of laughter. She said: "I thought smoking was meant to be a serious business." It is, and so is quitting. Being a smoker is also a very unpleasant business, but quitting doesn't have to be, and remember: I have only good news to give you.

If at times I appear to sound arrogant, or to belittle you, also remember I was the most stupid nicotine addict of all and have yet to meet one as badly hooked as I was. This conveniently leads me into the second warning. Daily I receive letters from satisfied users of Easyway saying something like:

"My son gave me your book three years ago and I stuck it in a drawer. I recently came across it, I don't even know why I read it because I had no intention of quitting. I wish I hadn't wasted three years."

Perhaps you are reading this book because someone who loves you doesn't want you to die. Perhaps you feel that now isn't the right time, or that you cannot bear to think about life without your little crutch or pleasure. One of the snags of the book is this chicken and egg situation. If I could immediately transfer you into your mind and body to show you how you would feel in just a few weeks, that's all that I would need to do. You'd think: "Will I really feel this great?" And I don't just mean health-wise or energy-wise. I mean confidence-wise too.

In order to help you escape from the nicotine trap, I need first to dispel the illusions that you get some genuine crutch or benefit from smoking. At this stage you can feel worse off than when you started:

"I knew it was killing me and costing me a fortune but at least I thought I was getting some pleasure from smoking. Now you've taken even that away from me without explaining how you are going to make it easy to stop."

The danger is to get halfway through the book and for panic to set in:

"My God! If I go on reading this I'm going to have to quit!"

The temptation is to stop reading, to put off the evil day. I've said that the nicotine trap is the most ingenious, subtle and sinister illusion that nature and mankind have ever combined to create. One of the major subtleties is that it is designed to make you put off the evil day.

You need to be aware of this. Even if you do feel a bit anxious, remember you have nothing to lose. If by the end of the book I haven't convinced you, then you don't have to quit. You can go on smoking with a clear conscience. But please, please don't deprive yourself of the chance to be free. I promise you that if you complete the book by the time we get to the ritual of the final cigarette, you'll be like a dog straining at the leash, impatient to be free. Now let's start to dispel some of these illusions:

SMOKERS CHOOSE TO SMOKE

5

SMOKERS CHOOSE TO SMOKE

Do they? Think back, when did you choose to become a smoker? Don't misunderstand me. I don't mean what was the date or the occasion of your first experimental cigarette. What I'm asking is when did you actually sit down and decide that you'd like to be a smoker for life? The vast majority of smokers when asking themselves that question soon realize that they never actually decided to become smokers. In fact, the story for the vast majority of smokers is almost identical. Does your own experience fit the pattern?

"This friend (relative, colleague whatever) kept offering me cigarettes. Eventually I tried one. It tasted awful but I sensed that my friend needed someone to smoke with so I kept on taking them. I can remember thinking: how can he keep smoking these filthy things, let alone pay good money for them? I thought I was doing him a favour. Then one day I asked him for a cigarette. He said it's time you bought a packet. I'd promised myself that I would never waste good money on them, but he was quite right, so I bought a packet and I've been buying them ever since. In fact now I have to have cigarettes all the time and start to get anxious even with the thought of running out."

Some smokers actually claim that they made the conscious decision to become hooked.

"Oh I decided to take up smoking because I was overweight."

We accept such explanations because we have been brainwashed since birth to believe that smoking actually helps to reduce weight. But even if that were true, to deliberately become addicted to Western society's No 1 killer disease in order to lose weight, is about as rational as sawing off one of your legs in order to lose weight. Surely a more rational solution would be not to eat so much or to change your diet.

In the UK fewer than 100 people per year die from heroin. Over 2,000 die every week from smoking. Yet we get very uptight about heroin addiction. The thought of one of our children getting hooked on heroin fills us with horror. In law a heroin addict is a criminal, yet not only is smoking legal, our own Treasury has the biggest vested interest, making hundreds of billions annually from the misery of smokers and permitting the tobacco industry to spend tens of millions per annum on promotion. Yet even in today's slightly more enlightened society, the general attitude is to regard smoking as a slightly disgusting and anti-social habit that might harm your health.

The only reason that any of us gets hooked is because of the influence of the millions of smokers who are already doing it. Yet they warn us not to do it. The ingenious subtlety that springs the trap is that cigarettes taste awful. If those first cigarettes tasted wonderful, alarm bells would ring. We'd think:

"Now I understand why my father coughs up his lungs every morning. No way am I going to fall into that trap."

But because they taste so awful, we are convinced that we couldn't get hooked. The really stupid thing is that we work so hard to get hooked or to inhale without coughing or feeling sick. Then we spend the rest of our lives, at odd times trying to rationalize why we do it, at other times trying to quit and eventually telling our own children not to be stupid just like our own parents tried to tell us.

In the UK the average 20-a-day smoker spends £100,000 (US$165,000) in their lifetime on cigarettes. A veritable fortune. Yet strangely, even the majority of smokers who can't afford to smoke claim that the money doesn't bother them.

Why doesn't it bother them? It wouldn't be so bad if we just set fire to that money. On second thoughts I suppose that is exactly what we do. But we also use it to risk awful diseases.

OK, most of us block our minds to those risks, our attitude tending to be either: "It won't happen to me", or "I'll quit before it does". But even if we are lucky enough not to contract one of the killer diseases, we suffer a lifetime of bad breath, lethargy, shortage of breath, coughing and wheezing and the filth and stigma.

The sheer slavery of being a smoker never seems to dawn on us. We smoke the vast majority of our cigarettes without even thinking about it. When we are allowed to smoke, we take cigarettes for granted. When we do consciously think about smoking we wish we hadn't started. We spend the other half of our lives feeling miserable and deprived in situations where we aren't allowed to smoke. What sort of hobby or pleasure is it, that when you are allowed to do it, you wish you didn't and only when you are not allowed to do it does it appear to be so precious?

It is a lifetime of being despised by the rest of the population. However, the very worst aspect of being a smoker is that otherwise intelligent, healthy, attractive human beings spend a lifetime despising themselves: every Budget day, every cancer scare, every time you get a cough, asthma or bronchitis, every time your family or friends give you that haunted look, every time you are not allowed to smoke or you are the lone smoker in the company of non-smokers, you have that awful sense of feeling unclean and stupid.

Before you became hooked on nicotine, you didn't need to smoke. You could enjoy social occasions, you could handle stress and you were perfectly happy without cigarettes. Do you really believe that anyone would actually choose the life that I have just described?

If you are in doubt, re-read from the beginning of this chapter. While you do so, remember the fourth instruction: keep an open mind.

The biggest idiot on the planet wouldn't choose to become a smoker, let alone a rational intelligent human being, and that's what the majority of smokers are. The smoking trap is a fascinating subject once you understand it. But until you do, everything appears to be topsy-turvy, back to front or upside-down. Ironically, the smokers that admit to being stupid are, in fact, intelligent and the smokers that try to convince you that smoking isn't stupid are stupid.

I've often been in the company of smokers who wax lyrical about the pleasures of being a smoker. I ask them:

"Do you encourage your children to smoke?"

"Of course not."

"Why not? You have just spent an hour telling me the immense crutch and/or pleasure you get from smoking. Why don't you want your children to share those delights?"

The smoker looks at me with astonishment. He thinks it's me who is being stupid. It doesn't seem to dawn on him that it's him. There's not a parent in western society that likes the thought of their children becoming hooked, and whether they be smokers or non-smokers, they cannot hide their pride if their children are non-smokers. This really means that the smoking parents wish they hadn't become hooked themselves!

There's not a smoker past or present that actually chose to become a smoker. Do you really believe that alcoholics choose to become alcoholics, or that heroin addicts actually choose to become addicted to heroin?

Unless you can accept that you didn't actually choose to become a smoker, there is little point in your reading on. However, you might argue, as some smokers do, that although you wish you hadn't lit that first cigarette, having gone through the considerable effort required in order to enjoy the taste and satisfaction of smoking tobacco, in spite of the health risks and the expense, you do choose to continue to smoke.

Now suppose I inform you that there is no plus side. Let me make myself quite clear: I do not mean that the disadvantages of being a smoker far outweigh the advantages – all smokers know that throughout their lives. I mean there are no advantages whatsoever; they are just illusions.

Supposing I were able to convince you that not only are there no advantages to being a smoker whatsoever, that not only doesn't smoking relieve boredom or stress, or assist relaxation and concentration, but does the complete opposite! That not only does it not give you courage and confidence but that the worst aspect of being a smoker is that it destroys your courage, your confidence and your self-respect. Would you still choose to continue smoking? If the answer is 'yes', I suggest we stop wasting each other's time. Let me tell you about what happened to me on 15th July 1983:

THE MIRACLE

6

THE MIRACLE

Imagine being fascinated by Egyptian hieroglyphs, spending your whole lifetime studying the subject but finding it completely incomprehensible and finally giving up even trying to solve the mysteries. Then by chance you discover the clue that breaks the code. Try to imagine the elation you would feel. Imagine how much more elated you would feel if your very life had depended on solving the mystery.

Can you imagine how the Count of Monte Cristo must have felt when he realized that he had finally escaped from that prison? That's how I felt when I discovered the clue that exposed the subtle mysteries of nicotine slavery and enabled me to escape. Can you begin to imagine how that elation was multiplied with the knowledge that I had the key that would enable every other smoker to escape?

What was that clue? It was contained in a medical pamphlet that my son gave to me. He knew that I was trying to quit and thought it might help. I don't even know why I read it and even when I did it was gobbledegook. For some reason I read it again and again. It was rather like one of those picture patterns where, if you stare at them long enough, suddenly, from out of the monotonous pattern, a fascinating picture is projected.

Gradually I was able to see behind the medical jargon and the gobbledegook, to remove the cobwebs and the chaff from the wheat. This is what was projected:

"Nicotine, a colourless, oily compound, is the drug contained in tobacco that addicts smokers. It is the fastest addictive drug known to mankind, and it can take just one cigarette to become hooked.

"Every puff on a cigarette delivers, via the lungs to the brain, a small dose of nicotine that acts more rapidly than the dose of heroin the addict injects into his veins. If there are twenty puffs for you in a cigarette, you receive twenty doses of the drug with just one cigarette.

"Nicotine is a quick-acting drug, and the levels in the blood stream fall quickly to about half within thirty minutes of smoking a cigarette and to a quarter within an hour of finishing a cigarette. This explains why most smokers average about twenty per day. As soon as the smoker extinguishes the cigarette, the nicotine rapidly starts to leave the body and the smoker begins to suffer withdrawal symptoms. Within seven seconds of lighting a cigarette fresh nicotine is supplied and the craving ends, resulting in a feeling of relaxation and confidence that the cigarette gives to the smoker."

Perhaps my extraction of the wheat from the chaff doesn't give you any wonderful revelations. But I had spent the previous third of a century wandering through a misty, nightmare world of lethargy, fear and depression and I believed that I could never escape from that world. It was as if I had suddenly awakened from that nightmare and found myself back in a real world of sunshine, health and freedom.

You could be forgiven for believing that I exaggerate. I assure you, I do not. It never ceases to amaze me that, apart from the health aspect, society's concepts about the subject of smoking are the complete opposite of the truth. It would be logical to believe that chain-smokers enjoy smoking more than casual smokers. It is a fallacy. When you chain-smoke even the illusion of pleasure has gone. I would lie in bed every night praying that I would wake up the next morning either having lost the desire to smoke or having acquired the will-power to quit. I knew smoking would soon kill me, but even then I couldn't quit.

Why was I so elated? Because I'd solved the mysteries of the nicotine trap. There was no flaw in my character that meant I could not enjoy life or cope with stress without smoking and there was no genuine pleasure or crutch in smoking. The whole filthy business was just an ingenious, sinister confidence trick. As with all confidence tricks, intelligent people will fall for them, but if you know something is a confidence trick, even a fool will not fall for it.

Smoking is like wearing tight shoes just to get the pleasure of taking them off. Before we start smoking, we don't need cigarettes to enjoy life or handle stress. But when we smoke that first cigarette, we put nicotine into the body. When we extinguish it the nicotine starts to leave, which creates an empty insecure feeling, the feeling that smokers learn to know as needing something to do with their hands or needing a cigarette.

If you light another cigarette the nicotine is immediately replaced, the empty insecure feeling disappears and is replaced by a feeling of relaxation, or satisfaction or whatever the smoker likes to describe it as. The 'buzz' is something else.

Of course, once you extinguish the second cigarette, the nicotine again starts to leave, the insecure feeling returns and you need another cigarette. This is why there is a chain reaction to smoking. I enjoy eating lobster, but I don't get into a panic when I can't have one and if I never ate another lobster in my life it wouldn't bother me. It also explains why the average 20-a-day smoker confesses that of the 20 they only actually enjoy one or two but still smoke the ones they don't enjoy.

From hereon I will refer to that empty feeling of wanting a cigarette as:

THE LITTLE MONSTER

7

THE LITTLE MONSTER

All smokers light their first experimental cigarettes for stupid reasons. Usually it's just curiosity or peer pressure. The reason doesn't really matter because they didn't need to smoke before they started and whatever their reason was, if they knew that they would become hooked, they wouldn't smoke the first one.

The only reason any smoker continues to smoke is not because they think it's cool or adult, not because they need something to do with their hands or need oral satisfaction, not because it relieves boredom or stress, not because it assists relaxation and concentration, but for one reason and one reason alone:

TO FEED THE LITTLE NICOTINE MONSTER

It is essential that you understand this. It is not an actual living monster inside your body, but its effect is exactly the same and I would like you to imagine that from the moment you fell into the nicotine trap you created this monster. Imagine it as a living tapeworm inside your body that you have been feeding and nurturing and which will eventually kill you unless you starve it. That is exactly what you are going to do.

I used to call myself a golf addict. That was because I loved playing golf and wanted to play more and more. I also used to refer to myself as a nicotine addict, not because I enjoyed it but because I used to smoke so much. But I never actually thought of smoking as drug addiction.

I've referred to the little monster. How can I describe a monster that ruins the lives of so many people and that currently causes the early death of over 3,500,000 smokers every year as little? Because although nicotine is the most powerful drug known to mankind in the speed that it hooks you – just one cigarette will do it, particularly if you have been a smoker before – fortunately you are never badly hooked. This is one of the subtleties of nicotine addiction, the actual physical withdrawal symptoms are so mild as to be almost imperceptible.

If that is true, why do smokers find it so difficult to quit and why do they suffer

THOSE TERRIBLE WITHDRAWAL SYMPTOMS?

8

THOSE TERRIBLE WITHDRAWAL SYMPTOMS

I've been a very lucky man and have had many exciting and exhilarating experiences in my life. One stands out head and shoulders above the rest:

THE MOMENT OF REVELATION

This is the moment when you know you are going to be free. I knew I was going to be free, but I wasn't expecting it to be easy and at the time I didn't realize that I was already free. Remember, I'd had many attempts to quit before and knew I had first to go through a period of misery. Amazingly there was no misery. I felt free even before I'd extinguished the final cigarette and that feeling of elation has never left me. I don't mean that my life is one continuous round of honey and roses. All people have good days and bad days, whether they be non-smokers, smokers or ex-smokers. If cigarettes genuinely created pleasure and relieved stress, smokers' lives would be all honey and roses and you would have no need to read this book. But whether I'm having a good day or a bad day, I know that the day would be less good or more miserable if I were still a smoker.

It wasn't until I looked back on those previous attempts and tried to remember where it hurt me that it dawned on me that there was no physical pain. Occasionally our failures at the clinics will engage in this kind of conversation:

"You said there's no pain. I've been going through agony."
"Describe the pain to me."
"It's awful, like flu."
"And your doctor diagnosed withdrawal from nicotine?"
"I haven't been to my doctor."
"Why not, it sounds like flu."

They haven't been to their doctor because they know that whatever they are suffering is not flu but a direct result of their attempt to quit. Ironically, if you said to a smoker, "You can have flu for five days after which you will be a happy non-smoker for the rest of your life," he would jump at the opportunity. Even when we have genuine flu, we feel physically awful, but no matter how bad we feel we can cope with the situation.

However, if you press smokers who are trying to quit to be more specific about the pain they are suffering, they come out with statements such as:

"I keep breaking out in a sweat." or
"I can't concentrate or sleep at night."

We point out to them that athletes break into a sweat every time they perform and that we all have periods when we can't concentrate or sleep at night. We don't seem to regard such things as a great tragedy, so where's the problem? They find it difficult to explain.

Don't misunderstand me. I know better than most people about the traumas that smokers suffer when trying to quit by using will-power. The point I'm making is that the torture is not physical. We believe that we suffer from nicotine withdrawal when we try to quit. No, we suffer from nicotine withdrawal throughout our smoking lives and it is only those withdrawal symptoms that make us want to light the next cigarette.

Many smokers find it difficult to understand this concept completely. However, it is absolutely essential that you do. Possibly the easiest way is to compare smoking with:

EATING

9

EATING

Imagine you are God and that you have created this incredible range of species. However, none of them will survive unless they eat. How do you make sure they eat? It's easy for us; our parents can explain why we must eat. But how do you ensure that wild animals eat? You equip them with an ingenious device called hunger. Some people believe that we eat because food tastes good. No, the true reason we eat is to end the aggravation called hunger. This is why the French wish you a good appetite rather than good food before a meal. It is true that we would rather satisfy our hunger with certain types of food than others, just as smokers would rather satisfy their craving for nicotine with their favourite brand, but just as they would rather smoke old rope than not at all, so a starving man will eat a rat.

If taste had anything to do with it smokers would never smoke more than one cigarette. In fact smokers will often switch to a brand that they dislike, or to cigars or a pipe, in the hope that this will help them to quit. All that happens is that, provided you persist long enough, you will acquire a taste for the new brand, cigar or pipe.

Some smokers believe that as youngsters they deliberately learned to inhale and acquire the taste. Not so. This would mean that they had planned to get hooked. We've already established that the biggest idiot on earth doesn't plan to get hooked. It works the other way around. The first cigarette creates the hunger; we only persevere and acquire the taste in order to satisfy the little monster.

Put yourself in the place of the Creator again. You've created this incredible variety of life. You've equipped each individual with hunger to ensure that it eats and survives. But how does it know the difference between food and poison? Again it's easy for human beings. If our parents are responsible, they'll ensure that any poisonous substances are safely locked away out of harm's way until we're old enough to be taught the difference between food and poison. But how do wild animals know the difference between food and poison?

A clever way would be to make food smell and taste good and to make poisons smell and taste awful. That's exactly what the creator and/or evolution did. Fortunately most smokers can remember how foul that first cigarette was. If you tried to inhale, the reason it made you cough and feel giddy and sick is because your body was saying:

YOU ARE FEEDING ME POISON! PLEASE STOP DOING IT!

The tobacco plant is, in fact, a cousin of deadly nightshade and contains several poisonous compounds including nicotine. Nicotine is one of the most powerful poisons known to mankind. It is commonly used as an insecticide. If you were to inject the nicotine content of just one small cigar directly into your vein, it would kill you. Please don't try it out. A student did some time ago. He died.

When you are learning to smoke, all you are actually doing is teaching your brain and body to become immune to the foul effects. It's rather like working on a farm. To start with, the animals smell awful, but eventually you become immune to their smell, and incidentally, they become immune to yours. The human body is an incredibly sophisticated machine. It will warn you when you feed it poison and if you are stupid enough not to heed that warning and continue to regularly feed poison, it will try to protect you. Rasputin was able to survive a dose of arsenic twenty times the size of the dose that would kill an average human being purely by gradually building a resistance to the poison.

Let's get back to the similarity between eating and smoking. We think of hunger as a rather unpleasant experience. The truth is that it is an incredibly ingenious device. I should emphasize that I'm not talking about starvation now, but the everyday business of enjoying three meals a day.

When we eat it's rather like filling up our car with fuel. We've provided our body with the energy and minerals it needs to survive. The moment we finish that meal we start to use up that energy but we don't immediately feel hungry again, unless, of course, we have dietary problems. In fact, if we get into a regular habit of eating, say, three meals a day, we need never even be aware of the aggravation called hunger, provided that we eat when our next meal is due and our body says to our brain, "Hey, I'm hungry, let's eat". You can then obtain the genuine pleasure of satisfying that hunger without being aware of any aggravation.

However, supposing, for whatever reason, that meal is not available. Now you suffer. I remember as a boy on Sundays we ate lunch at 2pm when my father returned from having a drink with his friends. The problem was the rest of the week we ate lunch at midday and my body and brain were geared up to eat then. Even 50 years later, as I write I, can smell that roast lamb, mint sauce, garden peas and roast potatoes. I can remember the agony, the absolute torture of those two hours. Now we've all experienced similar occasions at various times in our lives. But what physical pain do we actually undergo at such times? OK, our stomachs might be rumbling, but there's no actual physical pain. Nevertheless, it is physical, and we musn't underestimate its effect. Imagine having an itch on the tip of your nose and not being allowed to scratch it. That could drive you to distraction in just a few minutes.

How would you describe hunger? There's no physical pain. We can only describe it as an empty, insecure feeling that we know will only be satisfied by food. The feeling itself isn't so bad – just like the itch, it's not being allowed to satisfy it or scratch it that's the torture.

How do you describe the craving for nicotine? Are you in physical pain? No, you have just an empty, insecure feeling which you know will be satisfied by a cigarette. Just like a hunger for food, provided your brain is not aware of it, you do not suffer one iota, and provided when you do become aware of it, you are allowed to light up and relieve the empty, insecure feeling, you get genuine pleasure and relaxation. Except that it isn't genuine but simply:

AN INGENIOUS SUBTLE CONFIDENCE TRICK

It is this similarity to eating that fools us into believing that we get some genuine crutch or pleasure from smoking. With both, most of the time we are not even aware of the empty, insecure feeling. Once we are aware of it, providing we are allowed to imbibe food or nicotine, we immediately replace the empty, insecure feeling with a feeling of confidence, security and satisfaction.

That is one of the many ingenious subtleties of the nicotine trap. Although smoking and eating appear to be similar, in fact they are diametrically opposed. Hunger is a craving for food. Food is vital for health, energy, enjoyment, longevity and survival. Smoking is a craving for a deadly poison guaranteed to ruin your health, make you breathless and lethargic, make you miserable, shorten your life and kill you. The actual process of ending your hunger for food is genuinely pleasant. Good food does taste pleasant and, provided you are hungry and eating good food, the whole ritual is a tremendously pleasant experience. Whereas to relieve your craving for nicotine, you have to breathe obnoxious, poisonous fumes into your lungs. That is very unpleasant. If you haven't yet absorbed that message, then before you read any further, inhale cigarette after cigarette until you realize that breathing poisonous fumes into your lungs is decidedly unpleasant.

But the most important difference between eating and smoking is this: eating doesn't create a hunger for food. On the contrary it genuinely satisfies it. Not permanently, but that's even better: we can and do get the genuine pleasure of satisfying our hunger for food for the whole of our lives. Whereas smoking, far from ending the empty, insecure feeling of craving nicotine, not only causes it – we don't need cigarettes before we start smoking – but ensures that we suffer it for the rest of our lives.

Smokers often say to me: how can you possibly say that there is no genuine pleasure or crutch in smoking and at the same time admit that when a smoker lights a cigarette he genuinely feels more relaxed or less nervous than he did before he lit it? I reply:

"Do you think wearing tight shoes is relaxing?"

"Of course not."

"But you can't deny it is relaxing to remove tight shoes."

"I don't get the point."

"Just as if you hadn't worn tight shoes, you couldn't have got the pleasure of removing them, so if you hadn't lit the first cigarette, you wouldn't have had the need to relieve the empty feeling it created by lighting another one. That second cigarette didn't cure the empty feeling, it simply put more nicotine into your body. The first cigarette caused the problem. The other cigarettes, far from relieving it, just continued the problem."

There are many pathetic aspects to smoking. However, I think that the most pathetic aspect of all is that the real reason why smokers spend a small fortune risking awful diseases for a lifetime of lethargy, filth, loss of self respect and slavery is:

TO FEEL LIKE A NON-SMOKER

Am I telling you that the only reason that smokers smoke is to feel like a non-smoker? That is exactly what I'm telling you. But surely the mere statement is a contradiction. Not so. No one would question that it is relaxing to remove tight shoes. But what are you actually enjoying? The ending of the aggravation of wearing tight shoes. In other words, returning to the blissful state you were in before you put on tight shoes. What you are actually enjoying is:

FEELING LIKE A NON-TIGHT-SHOE-WEARER

Before we start the nicotine chain we don't need cigarettes. When nicotine leaves our body it causes the empty, insecure feeling.

The moment you light a cigarette that empty feeling begins to disappear and you feel more relaxed or less distressed than a moment before. The actual pleasure or crutch that you are experiencing is returning to the blissful state that you had the whole of your life before you started the nicotine chain and will have again the moment you break that chain.

What I am actually telling you is that cigarettes do absolutely nothing for you at all. I don't mean the disadvantages of being a smoker outweigh the advantages. All smokers know that instinctively and that's why smoking parents hate the thought of their children getting hooked. What I mean is:

THERE IS NO PLEASURE OR CRUTCH IN SMOKING WHATSOEVER

Perhaps you find this knowledge a revelation. Perhaps it fills you with panic. After all, you already knew that smoking is stupid, but at least you felt you were getting some benefits to justify your stupidity and all I've done so far is to remove that saving grace without explaining how easy and enjoyable it is to quit. This is the stage when some smokers panic and don't finish the book. Please don't fall for that trap. Remember:

I HAVE NOTHING BUT GOOD NEWS FOR YOU

However, perhaps you still find it difficult to believe that the only reason smokers continue to smoke is to feed that little monster. Surely if it were as simple as that it would be so obvious. Don't underestimate the incredible ingenuity of the trap. There are several reasons why it is difficult to see through the confidence trick. The first is:

THE BIG MONSTER

10

THE BIG MONSTER

From birth we are literally bombarded daily with information telling us that smoking is cool, pleasurable, adult, helps us to relax and concentrate, relieves boredom and stress, gives us courage and confidence, is a friend and crutch. Why should we not believe it? Every time you watch a film when someone is about to be executed, what is their final request? A beautiful woman? A wonderful meal? No, it's always a cigarette. What is this actually telling us?

"The greatest pleasure on this earth, and/or the crutch I most need to help me through this terrible trauma, is a cigarette."

When you see a film with a husband waiting outside the maternity ward, he is chain-smoking. When the baby is born cigars are handed around. These situations are being repeated in real life. It is also true that from birth we have been advised that smoking is a filthy, disgusting habit that will hook us, cost us a fortune and shorten our lives.

Be that as it may, every time you see a smoker light up a cigarette, particularly if they are strong, attractive people like Clint Eastwood, or sophisticated, beautiful women like Marlene Dietrich or highly intelligent people like Bertrand Russell, what they are actually telling you is, in spite of the cost and health risks:

SMOKING IS ENJOYABLE

Even non-smokers believe that smokers get some pleasure or crutch from smoking. Their attitude is:

"Obviously there is some pleasure or crutch, but what you've never had you don't miss, and I can do without the bad side, thank you very much."

The point I'm making is that before we ever light our first cigarette, we've already been subjected to massive brainwashing expounding the pleasure and benefits that smokers enjoy. So when we actually fall into the nicotine trap ourselves and discover that we do actually feel more relaxed or less distressed after we light up, and that we

28

would find it easier to concentrate with a cigarette, why should we even question the fact? After all, we were warned, why should we be surprised when it turns out to be true?

At this point I need to define Brainwashing. My dictionary defines it as: "to force a person to reject old beliefs and accept new ones by subjecting him to great mental pressure." I'm somewhat peeved when a celebrity that I've helped to cure, appears on television and says:

"He was great. He brainwashed me into seeing how lovely it is to be free!"

Why does that peeve me? Because I don't brainwash people. My definition of brainwashing is: to force a person to believe something that isn't true. From birth we are brainwashed to believe that there is some pleasure or benefit to be obtained from smoking. It is an illusion and a lie. My method is the complete opposite to brainwashing. It's counter-brainwashing, to enable the smoker to see through the illusion and the lie.

The big monster is the brainwashing. It's not the chemical addiction itself that makes it difficult to quit, but the belief that we are being deprived of a genuine pleasure or crutch. Fortunately we can destroy the big monster before you even extinguish the last cigarette. But first we must explain the other reasons why it is so difficult to see through the nicotine trap. The brainwashing or big monster is the first. Another is the little monster:

THE EMPTY INSECURE FEELING

11

THE EMPTY INSECURE FEELING

The second reason that the confidence trick is so difficult to see through is that the little monster is so imperceptible that we don't even realize it's there. There is no physical pain. It's just an empty, insecure feeling. And the third reason is, that feeling is identical to normal hunger and normal stress.

Smokers only ever light up during periods of stress. That might appear to be a contradiction. You might argue that one of the favourite cigarettes for most smokers is at a time of relaxation: after a meal. How many meals have you had in your life? Can you actually remember smoking all those cigarettes that you smoked after a meal? Did you sit there thinking, "This tastes really gorgeous"? Remember I've asked you to open your mind. Isn't it true that it's not so much that smokers enjoy smoking after a meal, as that they can't enjoy the occasion without smoking?

The point I'm making is that whether smokers are in a genuinely stressful situation, or in a situation like a meal or a party that would be completely enjoyable and relaxing for a non-nicotine addict, such situations would be stressful for nicotine addicts unless they can relieve the stress created by the little monster.

So, no matter what the occasion is, be it relaxing or stressful, immediately the smoker lights up they do actually feel more relaxed or less distressed than a moment before and their brain is fooled into believing that they have received a genuine crutch or pleasure.

The fourth reason why it is so difficult to see is that it happens so slowly and gradually that we don't realize it is happening to us. In my book *The Easy Way to Lose Weight* I point out that if overnight we awoke 30 pounds heavier with a grotesque belly, we'd rush off to our doctor in a panic wondering what awful disease we'd contracted. Our doctor then says:

"Don't worry, it looks disastrous but fortunately there is an easy cure; all you have to do is start eating the right foods."

Even if those foods tasted awful, we'd be quite happy to take our medicine. By the time you have finished this book, you will know that I love analogies. A Scottish client recently sent me a postcard thanking me for my help. He said that if you put a frog into boiling water it will immediately jump out. But if you put a frog into warm water and gradually bring it to the boil, the frog will happily remain in the water until it boils to death.

I emphasize that I don't know whether this is fact. I've no intention of putting it to the test and I'd rather that you didn't either. However, it is an excellent analogy. Possibly the most ingenious aspect of any addiction is that it happens so slowly and gradually that we aren't even aware that it is happening. Because the first cigarettes taste so awful, we are convinced that we couldn't get hooked. Because that empty, insecure feeling is almost imperceptible and identical to normal hunger and stress, we aren't even aware of it, and because in the early days our intake of tobacco is little and far between, for most of the time we are not smoking and we regard that state as normal.

However, the fifth and most powerful reason why we are fooled is that it works back to front. It's when we are not smoking that we suffer the empty, insecure feeling and when we light up we do actually feel more relaxed or less distressed than a moment before. We don't understand why. We don't need to understand why. We don't understand how eating satisfies hunger, or how scratching an itch seems to help, or why when we press the light switch the bulb lights up. We don't need to know how, all we need to know is it does.

It is the combination of these same five factors that makes all drug addiction appear difficult to kick. Because we suffer the empty insecure feeling when we aren't smoking, we don't blame the cigarette. Because the feeling is partially relieved the moment we light up, our brain is fooled into believing that the cigarette is giving confidence rather than destroying it. Imagine a heroin addict without heroin: the misery, the panic, the fear. Now picture the marvellous state of relief when finally he gets his fix and can plunge a needle into his vein. Can you imagine that?

Advanced heroin addicts believe they get a genuine pleasure from plunging a needle into their veins, whereas most people regard injections as anathema. Non-heroin addicts don't get into a panic when they can't get heroin. Society taught me to believe that heroin addicts take heroin for the marvellous highs they receive and then become addicted. Does that seem logical to you?

Let me tell you how to tell the difference between genuine highs and drug addiction. Genuine highs, like Christmas or watching a good film, are a pleasure not a need. Genuine highs are enjoyed at the time, but you don't necessarily feel deprived and miserable afterwards. Genuine highs can be taken or left, but with drug addiction, the addict is forced to repeat the process, even when that process involves sticking a hypodermic syringe into a vein or breathing obnoxious fumes into their lungs.

Heroin addicts don't stick needles into their veins to get highs, they do it to try to relieve the awful lows that the previous doses created. Smokers breathe obnoxious and toxic fumes into their lungs for exactly the same reason: to try to relieve the empty, insecure feeling that the first cigarette started. Do you envy heroin addicts? Of course not. On the contrary you pity them. That's how non-smokers regard you when you breathe those cancerous fumes into your lungs. Society has a misconception that youngsters start smoking because they believe it's cool. They don't. All youngsters instinctively hate smoking until they get hooked. We only assume they think it's cool because we can't understand why they do it. Neither can they and neither did you. Is it cool to inject yourself with heroin or to get your foot caught in a bear trap? Of course not. Before you got hooked you saw smokers not as cool but stupid. If you follow all the instructions, very soon you'll be looking at other smokers not with envy, but with genuine pity as you would look at a heroin addict. The only mystery will be trying to figure out why you ever needed to do it and wondering why you cannot convince your smoking friends and relatives:

HOW NICE IT IS TO BE A NON-SMOKER AND HOW EASY IT IS TO BECOME ONE

This book is entitled *Allen Carr's Easy Way To Stop Smoking*. Perhaps you are wondering why I don't just get on and explain the easy way to stop. I understand your frustration. Please bear with me. It will help if I explain the analogy of:

THE MAZE

12

THE MAZE

Imagine yourself as a youngster wandering into a beautiful garden so magnificent that you decided to remain there. After a while you begin to suspect that the exotic plants, beautiful as they might appear, are giving off toxic fumes that are beginning to affect your health. So you decide to leave the garden. However, leaving is not as simple as it first appears; in fact the garden turns out to be an incredibly complicated and ingenious maze. Let's assume that the maze has 20 junctions and at each junction you have two choices. Let's also assume that every time you make the wrong choice, you eventually find yourself back in the centre of the maze. Let's assume that you have average luck: that you make the right choice every other time. It would take you ten attempts to escape from the maze.

I explained in Chapter 2 how smokers are imprisoned as effectively as if they were surrounded by iron bars. Assume that, on average, smokers make a serious attempt to quit once in every three years. On average, it would take you 30 years to escape from the maze. If you can understand the analogy, it explains why it takes most of us so long to escape from the nicotine trap and, tragically, why one in two smokers do not live long enough to escape.

However, supposing you had a map of the maze, which indicated the correct turn to take at each junction. Provided you followed all the instructions implicitly, you would find it easy to escape from the maze.

EASYWAY IS THAT MAP

But there are other maps, each giving contradictory information. Who can you trust? How do you know which map is correct? This is why I can't just give you the instructions. Unless I can first convince you that I understand more about the nicotine trap than any other person on this planet and that mine is the only true map, why should you follow my instructions? This is the problem that has confronted me since I first discovered Easyway. Established medical professionals are widely accepted as the true experts on helping smokers to quit. It is true that they know more than I do about the health risks caused by smoking. But, frankly, they haven't the slightest idea how to escape from the prison. It is a fact that more people attending our clinics are from the medical profession than any other single profession.

The truth is, that apart from putting the fear of God into them, doctors have no idea about helping smokers to quit. Because they don't understand nicotine addiction, their attitude and the attitude of society generally is, "Try this. If that doesn't work, try that, try anything."

In 1998 I was invited to attend the 10th World Conference On Tobacco and Health, which I considered a golden opportunity to explain the Easyway method to an influential group. But I was introduced to the assembly almost with an apology: "This is the first time we have invited a commercial interest".

I'd always thought of myself as someone who was trying to free smokers from nicotine slavery and as I was giving the benefit of my knowledge to the whole world completely free of charge, I was somewhat shocked to be described as a commercial interest. However, I was delighted and honoured to have been invited. But the true irony was that practically the whole of the conference was sponsored and dominated by the nicotine replacement industry. Even the name is a misnomer: NRT is nicotine continuation not replacement, and there's nothing therapeutic about it either. Having sat through lecture after lecture listening to these medical experts desperately searching for a solution to the devastation caused by nicotine addiction, at last I had the opportunity to inform them that I had the simple solution to their problem. Amazingly, the vast majority of these dedicated people, who had spent many years trying to solve the problem, couldn't be bothered to turn up. The few that did, far from being appreciative, were actually aggressive.

Now you might conclude that, as I'm not a qualified doctor, these dedicated professionals regarded my method as not worthy of investigation. However, I would ask you to consider these two unarguable facts. If the incredible influence and combined power of the established medical profession had the solution, why would I even need to write this book? I'm just one isolated individual. If I hadn't got the solution, why would I be widely regarded as the 'stop smoking' guru? There is only one reason:

MY SYSTEM WORKS!

Now I would refer you back to the list of questions in Chapter 4. At the conference I prepared a similar list consisting of 23 questions. On average, these medical experts got 17 out of the 23 wrong, about 75 percent. Who am I to say I was right and they were wrong? This is what this book is about. I need to explain the reasons for my instructions. You will be the judge. I rely on your intelligence. Incidentally, so do you, so make sure you come to the correct solution. However, if I am right, and you are relying on the advice given by the medical experts, at three out of every four of the junctions that you come to in the maze, your map is giving you the wrong turn. Is it surprising that smokers find it so difficult to escape? With the correct map it's easy to quit. Let me make it quite clear. It is easy to quit. That is a fact. Just think for a moment:

WHY SHOULD IT BE DIFFICULT TO QUIT SMOKING?

13

WHY SHOULD IT BE DIFFICULT TO QUIT SMOKING?

Nobody forces us to smoke but ourselves, so if you decide that you never want to smoke again, why should it be difficult? The so-called experts usually give two answers to that. The first we have already discussed in Chapter 8: those terrible withdrawal symptoms from nicotine.

Nicotine may be the most powerful drug known to mankind in the speed that it hooks its victims – why else would over 90 percent of adult males in western society be hooked a few decades ago? – but fortunately you are never badly hooked on the drug itself. In fact, after just three weeks of abstinence, the little monster dies and you will no longer suffer the empty, insecure feeling of the body craving nicotine.

Now, I'm aware that the thoughts of abstaining for just an hour will drive many smokers into panic. In fact, this fear prevents some smokers from ever attempting to quit. There are other smokers in whom, when they try to quit, the attempt creates such panic that they actually smoke their next cigarette quicker than if they hadn't tried to quit.

But have no fear. Although that panic feeling may be triggered by the little monster, it is actually caused by the big monster – the brainwashing. Fortunately, you don't have to abstain at all in order to kill the big monster. We are going to do that before you extinguish that final cigarette. That is one of the reasons I want you to continue to smoke in the meantime.

A smoker at one of my early clinics said:

"I might as well tell you at the start, I really resent having to seek your help. I know I'm a strong-willed person. I'm in control of everything else in my life, but I can't quit smoking. If only I could smoke while I was quitting, I'm sure I could succeed."

This sounds contradictory, but I know what he meant. We believe quitting smoking is a very difficult and stressful exercise. What is our crutch during periods of difficulty and stress? A cigarette. At the very time we most need our crutch – we are deprived of it. That smoker didn't realize it at the time, and I must admit that it hadn't occurred to me either, but that is one of the ingenuities of Easyway – you can carry on smoking right up until the time you become a non-smoker.

The other reason why I want you to continue to smoke until the ritual of the final cigarette, is because it is only when you are not smoking that you crave a cigarette and get into a panic if you can't have one. That's when your brain will close your mind to all the logical reasons that you shouldn't smoke and desperately search for any flimsy excuse to allow you to continue to smoke, or to put off the evil day when you have to quit.

I don't want to be talking to the distorted, panicked mind of a drug addict. I want to talk to the same rational brain with which you would appraise other subjects.

All smokers have a permanent tug-of-war going on in their minds. Most of their smoking lives they try not to think about it. But it's permanently there, like an ever increasing black cloud in your subconscious mind. On one side of the tug-of-war, the black side: it's filthy and disgusting, killing me, costing me a fortune and controlling my life. On the other side, the good side: it's my pleasure, my crutch.

There is no good side. Like all drug addiction it is a tug-of-war of fear. The good side isn't a pleasure or crutch, it's panic: how can I enjoy life or cope with life without cigarettes? Non-smokers don't suffer that panic. It was created by the first cigarette and perpetuated by every subsequent one. I knew cigarettes were killing me and costing me a fortune. Logically you would think that the fear of contracting lung cancer would outweigh the fear of quitting. But lung cancer is a fear of the future. It might never happen, or hopefully I'll quit before it does. Whereas if I quit today I have to cope with the fear of stopping now. Another ingenuity of the nicotine trap is to ensure we put off the evil day for as long as possible.

I thought health followed by wealth in that order would be the greatest gains that I would obtain if ever I managed to quit. Amazingly, when I did manage to quit, marvellous gains as they obviously are, neither of them came in the first three. One that did come in the first three was to be rid of that panic feeling. I think it's time to tell you about:

THE MAN ON THE YACHT

A few years ago the chief executive officer of a huge conglomerate sought my help. He said:

"I never wanted to be a smoker, I was a good athlete at school, but you know what it was like in the old days. If you were a man and didn't smoke, you were regarded as a cissy. But having spent all this money and ruined my health, I really resent society suddenly turning around and treating me like some sort of social leper and have resisted all the attempts of my family, friends and colleagues, either to frighten me, or to humiliate me into stopping smoking. My attitude to smoking is this: I don't kid myself that I get any advantages at all from smoking. I know I was missing nothing before I started and I can remember how hard I had to work to learn to smoke. As far as I am concerned, smoking is a disease that society inflicted on me as a youngster, but at my time in life, society is damn well stuck with me. If I want to smoke, I smoke, whether it be in the theatre or in the home of a non-smoker.

"But I was recently on holiday on the Mediterranean. I met another businessman who was head of an equally large firm. He offered to take me out deep-sea fishing. We started out at about 7am, just the two of us on the boat. We'd been going for about an hour. I was feeling really great. The sun had begun to rise and I was standing in my shorts breathing in the briny. I reached for a cigarette. I'd forgotten to bring any. In panic I turned to the other man and to my horror realized that he was not only a non-smoker, but one of those supercilious types that have to make their views known. I thought: 'I'll just have to suffer.' Half an hour later, I was pulling my hair out. I thought: 'This is ridiculous. I'm supposed to be enjoying myself.' I sauntered up to him and said: 'Look, old man, I've forgotten my cigarettes. If you don't have any on the boat, we'll have to go back.'"

Just think of the wording: "If you don't have any on the boat", as if it was the other man's fault. Why should he have any? He wasn't a smoker. The conversation continued:
"Go on, you're pulling my leg, you surely don't want to smoke out here?"
"I assure you I'm serious."
"Oh, come on, just breathe this air into your lungs. Can't you really go a few hours without one?'
"Look, if you want me to enjoy this trip, I need cigarettes."
"I can't understand it myself, but you are my guest and if you really are serious then we'll go back."

The narrative continued:
"It took an hour and a half to get back. I felt so stupid. I couldn't look at this other guy. I was just staring straight out to sea. But every now and again, out of the corner of my eye, I could see him staring up at me, wondering what sort of half-wit I was. I'm about six-four and the other guy must have been about five-eight. But every moment I was feeling shorter and shorter and more and more miserable. Then it suddenly hit me. Here I was, Managing Director of this conglomerate, no one pushes me around. Here I am resisting all the efforts of my family and friends to make me stop, being made to look a fool in front of this man. It finally occurred to me that it was the cigarettes that were controlling my life. It was as if all of my life I had been obsessed with turning a rusty tap to no avail, then suddenly realizing that it had a left-handed thread. I'd heard about your reputation, and I decided there and then that, after the holiday, I would fix an appointment to see you. But the nub of the story was, it took

us an hour and a half to get back. I got the cigarettes, in fact four packs. It took
another hour and a half to get back to where we were. I was so pleased with myself,
I didn't smoke a single cigarette the whole of the trip! It didn't even bother me. At the
end of the trip I thanked my host, but he refused to shake my hand. I said: 'Are you
annoyed that we went back?' He replied: 'Not in the least. You told me that you
needed them, we wasted hours getting them, and I've been watching you, you haven't
smoked a single cigarette!' "

Now, how do you explain that to a non-smoker? Every smoker on the planet knows
the panic that man felt when he suddenly discovered that he was in the middle of the
ocean with no cigarettes, and every smoker knows how proud he felt because he
didn't have to smoke them once he had them. You've probably already guessed that
the first thing he did when he left the non-smoker was to light a cigarette!

This story illustrates several important aspects about smoking, some of which I
will refer to later. But the one I wish you to concentrate on now is that the man only
suffered the panic feeling when he had no cigarettes. Once he had cigarettes the
feeling went, he didn't even need to smoke. If that feeling had been physical, it would
still have been there.

Don't misunderstand me. There is a physical effect when the body is deprived of
nicotine. The little monster does exist. But it is so slight most smokers have lived and
died without ever realizing that they suffered from it. If you observe smokers when
they haven't smoked for some time, they will either have their hands near their
mouths, or they will appear to be restless, or if everything else is still, they will be
grinding their teeth. I believe I ruined my teeth with this perpetual grinding. I didn't
relate it to smoking; I thought it was caused by the other stresses and strains of life.

The panic feeling is purely mental, caused by the big monster – the belief that we
cannot enjoy life or cope with life without a cigarette. Smokers can go all night
without a cigarette. Nowadays most smokers leave the bedroom before they light up.
Many have breakfast first. Some will even leave the house or arrive at their work
place before they light up. They've gone ten hours without a cigarette, but they aren't
climbing up the wall. But if they'd gone ten hours during the day without one, they
would be. If it were purely physical, it wouldn't matter if it were night or day.

Naturally, they will be anticipating that first cigarette with relish. However, if
when they went to light that cigarette, you had snatched it from their lips and taken
their packet, they would have broken your arm to get those cigarettes.

That panic feeling isn't physical. It starts before you even run out of cigarettes. You
must often have been in those situations when it's late at night, you do a mental
calculation: "I reckon I'll be up about another four hours, but I've only got about an
hour's supply left in the packet!" The seeds of panic are already sown. It's not quite so
bad when you are being entertained; you can always feign a headache and leave early.

However, if you are the host you are trapped. The panic reaches its height when you are actually smoking your last cigarette. Or even worse, when you have meticulously rationed those last few cigarettes.

Your guests finally take the hints that you have been blatantly broadcasting for the last two hours. You have two cigarettes left. One to smoke before you go to bed and that really essential one for the morning on which will depend whether you settle for a sleepless night, or spend two hours searching for an all-night garage. There is one other smoker in the company, one whose only contribution to the conversation throughout the evening has been to draw everyone else's attention to the number of cigarettes that you smoke, and to repeatedly enquire why you can't be like them and only smoke a few cigarettes a day?

All others present are gravely and silently nodding their agreement, except your non-smoking spouse, who finds it necessary to make regular interruptions of: "That's what I've been saying for years!" Why are they all oblivious to the fact that the so-called casual smoker has matched you cigarette for cigarette throughout the evening? Even more frustrating is that they are also oblivious to the fact that although that smoker generously arrived with two bottles of wine, they omitted to bring any cigarettes, and it's your cigarettes that they have been chain-smoking ever since the meal finished and that's why you only have two left and are beginning to panic. Then they drop a bombshell: "Do you mind if I have one of those?"

"Mind! Of course I mind! You can have a pint of my blood! I might even give you one of my kidneys! But there is no way you are having one of those cigarettes!" That is what we are thinking, but what do we do? We meekly hand over one of those precious cigarettes with "Of course", desperately hoping that our tone or expression didn't betray our true feelings. In case I'm now helping to bring on that panic feeling, let me remind you, the drug creates that feeling, non-smokers don't suffer it. Soon you'll be free of it.

I was discussing the two main reasons that the so-called experts attribute to why smokers find it so difficult to quit. One is the terrible withdrawal symptoms. I trust that I have adequately dealt with that one. The second reason they give is that:

SMOKING IS A HABIT

14

SMOKING IS A HABIT

I regard myself as a reasonably intelligent and inquisitive person. Having escaped from the nicotine trap, I find it incredible that for years I insipidly lapped up the clichés and platitudes of the so-called experts without even questioning them. Probably the most common and at the same time most stupid is:

YOU WON'T STOP UNLESS YOU REALLY WANT TO

These so-called experts make the statement as if they are revealing some profound insight into the mysteries of nicotine addiction. The statement is meaningless. Of course you won't stop unless you really want to. Why would you even make the attempt if you didn't want to quit?

The second most common and equally ridiculous platitude is:

SMOKING IS A HABIT AND HABITS ARE DIFFICULT TO BREAK

I can understand why smoking is commonly regarded as a habit. After all, there appears to be no other logical explanation. But are habits difficult to break? As an Englishman, all my life I've been in the habit of driving on the left side of the road. This causes some considerable inconvenience to Americans or Continentals who visit our islands. However, they are fortunate in that the vast majority of countries that they visit also drive on the right and they are not inconvenienced. The people that are most inconvenienced by their obsession to drive on the left are the people who do so.

Every time I visit the Continent or the States I'm forced to break the habit. Inconvenient it may be, but difficult it is not. I immediately break the lifetime's habit and when I return to England, I find it just as easy to return to the left. The truth is that we make and break habits every day of our lives.

The only reason why we believe habits are difficult to break is because the most common 'habit' that we would all really love to break is the smoking 'habit', and because most of us find it so difficult or even impossible to break it, we assume that habits are difficult to break. Now with a habit that kills us and costs us a fortune, when all we have to do to break it is to stop lighting cigarettes, why do we find it so difficult? Because it isn't habit:

IT IS DRUG ADDICTION

And one of the reasons that makes it difficult to quit is believing that it is habit and not drug addiction. Perhaps you fear that might make it even harder to quit. Not so. Once you understand it completely, it's easy to quit. The only reason we believe it's habit is because we cannot think of any rational reason to justify our stupidity. All our smoking lives we try to analyze why we smoke:

"I like the taste."
What has taste got to do with it? We don't eat cigarettes. In fact, tobacco is filthy and disgusting.
"I like the ritual."
Are you actually telling me you enjoy a ritual of spending a fortune to risk awful diseases and suffer a lifetime's slavery? If so, I'm afraid you really are stupid.
"But it's cool to have a burning cigarette in your mouth."
Then why not be even more cool and stick it in your ear? At least you won't have to breathe the cancerous fumes into your lungs.
"It gives me something to do with my hands."
You'll find a biro much healthier and a lot cheaper.
"Oh, that marvellous feeling of the smoke hitting my lungs!"
It's called suffocation. The worst aspect of smoking is that you have to choke yourself to do it.
"It's just oral satisfaction."

This is the Freud syndrome. The belief that we haven't been properly weaned and that the cigarette is no more than a dummy – a substitute for our mother's breast. I must admit that before I discovered the true reasons why I smoked, I did give some credence to this excuse; after all, it does have an element of logic to it. However, on closer scrutiny it is just as implausible as all the others.

The fact is that we are successfully weaned at an early age and, fortunately, for most of us, several years pass before we feel a desire to smoke cigarettes.

In truth, one of the factors that is helping smokers to quit nowadays is this belief that a cigarette is just a substitute for a dummy. If you had to suck a dummy in company you'd die with embarrassment, and if smoking were simply oral satisfaction you wouldn't have to set light to the cigarette. But smokers not only have to set light to them, they also have to inhale the filth into their lungs. Because that's how they get the nicotine. That's all they are really after:

THE NICOTINE

So after we've countered all the logical reasons for smoking, we are left with the only reason that appears logical, the reason that society has brainwashed us to believe – it's just habit, and habits are difficult to break. But even if this were true, it doesn't explain why, if the initial experimental cigarettes tasted foul, and we had no need to smoke before we got hooked, we worked so hard to acquire the habit. If, as most smokers admit, they only enjoy one or two a day, why do they smoke the others? And if the actual physical withdrawal pains from nicotine are almost imperceptible,

WHY DO SMOKERS FIND IT SO DIFFICULT TO QUIT?

15

WHY DO SMOKERS FIND IT
SO DIFFICULT TO QUIT?

Because they use the 'will-power' method. I define the 'will-power' method as any method that differs from Easyway. I define Easyway as a set of instructions which, if followed, will enable any smoker to quit immediately, permanently and easily, without using will-power, gimmicks or substitutes and without suffering withdrawal symptoms or weight gain.

Because the so-called experts do not understand the mysteries of drug addiction and therefore do not have an accurate map of the maze, their advice tends to be: try this, if it doesn't work try that, try anything as long as you keep trying. What I am about to say might appear to be arrogant. I make no apologies. I haven't got time for false modesty. We believe that it is intrinsically difficult to stop smoking. Therefore try anything that will make it easier. No, what I want you to see, and to help the rest of the world see, is that it is intrinsically easy to quit smoking. Easyway is a set of instructions that will enable any smoker to quit easily. So all other methods, whether you combine your own will-power with NRT, laser treatment, hypnosis, acupuncture or similar gimmicks, actually make it harder to quit. I do not dispute that millions of smokers have succeeded in quitting after using a variety of different methods. This just goes to confuse an already incredibly confused issue. They quit in spite of those methods not because of them.

Let us examine a typical attempt to quit smoking when using the 'will-power' method. The nicotine trap is not only ingenious in the manner that it springs the trap, but in keeping its victims trapped for the whole or most of their lives. Referring back to the analogy of the maze, for the first few years we actually believe that we are smoking because we choose to smoke and are in full control.

Over the years the gunge gradually accumulates inside our bodies and our health begins to decline both physically and mentally. At odd times in our lives, something will trigger an attempt to quit. We then take our heads out of the sand and weigh up the pros and cons of being a smoker. When we do this, we discover what we already knew:

SMOKERS ARE FOOLS!

Although we know that we'll be better off as non-smokers, providing we can achieve it, we do believe that we are making a genuine sacrifice. Quite why cigarettes are so precious, we are never sure. We just sense that during both good times and bad times, we seem to need them. It never seems to occur to us, that it's not so much that we enjoy them, but feel empty and insecure without them.

Although this need for a cigarette is an illusion, we have been successfully deluded. From birth we have been brainwashed to believe that smoking provides a genuine crutch or pleasure. Once we get hooked ourselves, the nicotine addiction confirms the illusion.

Added to this is the even more frightening brainwashing of how difficult it is to quit. There are endless stories of people like me that once quit for six months yet were still pulling their hair out. Complaining stoppers who have quit for 20 years yet are still craving the occasional cigarette. It's these complaining stoppers that convince us: once a smoker, always a smoker, you can never be completely free.

Even worse are the non-whingers who convince you that they no longer crave cigarettes and how lovely it is to be free. They raise your hopes. But next time you meet them, they are puffing away, and you think: "They must have missed them. Why else would they have started again?"

You've seen other smokers with hacking coughs, asthma, bronchitis or emphysema. It's obvious that they are getting no crutch or pleasure from smoking, yet they still puff away. Added to all this brainwashing you've probably been through similar experiences yourself.

So, instead of starting off the attempt to quit with a feeling of "EUREKA! Have you heard the wonderful news? I no longer need to punish my body or my pocket. I'm free! I'm a non-smoker!", we start with a feeling of doom and gloom as if we were making some terrible sacrifice and attempting the impossible, rather than being freed from slavery and the worst disease we are ever likely to suffer from.

Let's assume that we possess sufficient courage and will-power to abstain for a couple of hours or days. The problem is: once you stop smoking, all the powerful reasons that made you want to stop begin to dissipate. The congestion soon goes, we have more energy, more money and that holier-than-thou feeling of being free. The facts haven't changed, but the importance of those facts in our minds has. It's rather like seeing a bad accident when driving. That slows you down for a couple of miles, but the next time you are late for an appointment, you've forgotten about it.

So, the moment you extinguish what you hope will be your last cigarette, the powerful reasons that made you want to quit are rapidly disappearing and losing their effect. However, on the other side of the tug-of-war, the little nicotine monster hasn't been fed. There's no physical pain. In fact we only know the feeling as:

I WANT A CIGARETTE!

Our brains have worked out that there is not one logical reason why we should want a cigarette. But for some unknown reason we do. We are not aware that the feeling is just the death throes of the little monster. All we know is that for some illogical reason we want a cigarette. We also know that we musn't have one. If you want something and can't have it, you will feel deprived and miserable.

One of the times our brains are triggered to light a cigarette is when we are depressed and if we can't have one, we feel more depressed and the need to light that cigarette is even greater. It creates a chain reaction. In no time at all our minds are obsessed with but one thought: to find any flimsy excuse that will allow us to have just one cigarette.

I'm ashamed to admit it, but before I discovered Easyway, during my vain attempts to quit when using the 'will-power' method, I resorted to such tactics as banging my head against a wall hoping that my wife or children would say: "I can't bear to watch you suffering this torture, please start smoking again if you must." That was all I needed to hear. I could now start smoking again with dignity. It wasn't I who had failed. I was only smoking to please my family.

Perhaps you have also resorted to such histrionics in the past. It is quite common and this is what creates the illusion that smokers suffer terrible physical withdrawal symptoms when they try to quit. The physical pain is no worse than the tantrums of a child deprived of its chocolates. However, the mental anguish can be genuine torture.

The fact is, the moment your brain starts to say: "I want a cigarette", you have immediately switched from being a smoker who wanted to become a non-smoker, to a non-smoker who wants to become a smoker. Eventually the chain effect that I described above will wear down your resolution and will-power. Doubts will creep in. You'll start searching for reasons that will allow you to have just one cigarette: "I've got through five days. I deserve just one cigarette." After five days' abstinence that cigarette will probably taste weird. It might even taste foul. This gives you hope. You think: "Great! I'm getting off these things. I don't even like the taste now."

But taste has nothing to do with it. It never did. That little nicotine monster had been wandering through the desert for five days dying of thirst. That was the only reason that the big monster was saying: "I want a cigarette". When you lit that cigarette you kept that little monster alive. Not only did you keep it alive, but can you imagine how precious that drink was after five days? As I will explain later, cutting down doesn't help you to quit. On the contrary, it guarantees that you remain hooked for the rest of your life.

Once you've found the excuse to have just one cigarette, you soon discover that one cigarette isn't enough. The cigarette, far from becoming less precious, is now the most precious object on the planet. The next stage is usually to compromise: "I don't want to stop completely. So I'll just smoke five a day, or I'll just smoke on special occasions."

Before we know it we are smoking more than we did when we decided to quit. So do we decide to quit again? No, we simply change our excuses:

"It's my only pleasure in life."
Oh, come on. What about companionship, love, eating, friendship, energy, health or just the sheer joy of living?
"They tell you everything gives you cancer nowadays."
And do you meticulously search out all those carcinogens and make sure you get the lion's share?
"I could step under a bus tomorrow."
Yes, but I don't suppose you would be stupid enough to step under a bus deliberately. I presume like most people you go out of your way to avoid it.
"I believe car exhaust fumes are worse than smoking."
You could be right. But have you ever met anyone stupid enough to put their mouth over a car's exhaust pipe and breathe in the fumes?

The excuses to justify our failure to quit smoking are just as illogical as our excuses to smoke in the first place. A slightly more logical excuse is: "I picked the wrong time. I should have waited till after my holiday or after this or that stressful situation." But isn't there always some situation in the not too distant future which will allow us to put off the evil day?

Eventually you run out of excuses and reach the stage I got to: "I know I'm an idiot, but whether I like it or not, I just cannot enjoy life or handle life without my little crutch." I truly believed that, and because I believed it I was miserable when I wasn't allowed to smoke. I would give it my best shot, but in the end my will-power would run out. I could stand the misery no longer.

Like the man on the yacht, I knew instinctively that I was an idiot being a smoker. However, I took the attitude that I would rather have the shorter, sweeter life of the smoker than the longer, miserable life of the non-smoker. If that were the real choice, I wasn't actually being stupid, it was a perfectly rational decision to make and I would still be a smoker. Correction, I would be dead. I'm eternally grateful that it isn't true, and that not only have I already experienced the best 15 years of my life since I escaped, but look forward to many more.

Let's analyze exactly why the 'will-power' method makes it so difficult to succeed. We start the attempt with several distinct disadvantages. Because of the tug-of-war all smokers are schizophrenic throughout their smoking lives. Part of our brain wants to quit and part wants to continue to smoke. For most of our smoking lives the second part is in the ascendency. When the desire to quit becomes greater than the desire to continue, we decide to quit. However, the desire to continue doesn't disappear altogether. So we are not completely committed in the first place, and as I explained above, the moment you quit, and the longer you quit, the more your reasons for quitting dissipate.

We start our attempt with a feeling of sacrifice because we do believe that we get some genuine pleasure or crutch from smoking. That belief doesn't disappear just because we quit.

On the contrary, absence makes the heart grow fonder, and if you've ever suffered the misery of the 'will-power' method you'll know that, in no time at all, the most precious thing on earth is a cigarette.

We start the attempt by believing that quitting smoking is very difficult if not impossible. We also believe that it takes tremendous will-power and that, even if we possess sufficient will-power, we must first go through an indeterminate period of misery and deprivation.

Many smokers believe that you can never be completely free. I used to believe it. This is one of the difficulties of all drug addiction – it's negative. If you have a positive objective, like passing a driving test, once you've passed, the doubt is over. But if your object is not to do something for the rest of your life, how can you be sure that you've succeeded until you've lived the rest of your life? You are waiting not to smoke again, you are waiting to see if you fail and hoping that you never do.

I'm often asked: "When will I feel like a non-smoker?" In fact, smokers don't feel different from non-smokers. Oh, you'll have more energy and more confidence, but you won't feel a different person. Just think, when you extinguish a cigarette as a smoker, apart from the fact that you are no longer congesting your lungs, do you feel that you are a different person? It's rather like asking: "What does it feel like to be someone that doesn't eat bananas?" You can't answer that question. But re-phrase it: "What does it feel like to be someone that wants a banana but can't have one?" It feels lousy!

We also believe that, even if by some miracle we do succeed, life will never be quite as good. Meals will never be quite so enjoyable and it won't be so easy to answer that phone. It's not surprising smokers find it so difficult to quit when they use the 'will-power' method and that the majority of the ones that do spend the rest of their lives at odd times feeling they are missing out, envying smokers and trying to resist the occasional temptation. To me it's a miracle how any smokers manage to quit with the 'will-power' method and not surprising that so many get hooked again, even after years of abstinence.

With the 'will-power' method, you extinguish what you hope will be your final cigarette with a feeling of doom and gloom. You force yourself through a self-imposed trauma, like a child being deprived of its chocolates, hoping that, if you have the will-power to suffer the misery long enough, one day you'll wake up with the feeling:

EUREKA! I'M FREE!

Very few smokers that actually succeed in quitting when using the 'will-power' method ever experience the 'Moment of Revelation'. With Easyway every smoker can experience it. So:

HOW DOES EASYWAY MAKE QUITTING SO EASY?

16

HOW DOES EASYWAY MAKE QUITTING SO EASY?

It works in the exact opposite way to other methods in two important respects. First, it concentrates on the real problem – removing the need or desire to smoke, rather than patronizing smokers by telling them what they already know – it's killing you and costing you a fortune.

The other is that with the 'will-power' method we quit first and go through the trauma hoping to reach the 'Eureka' stage. For a few days the little monster wants feeding. This triggers the big monster to want a cigarette. There's no physical pain, the misery that we suffer is that we are not allowed to have a cigarette. It's like having an itch that you aren't allowed to scratch. We don't even realize that the little monster exists. We believe our desire for the cigarette is because we are making a genuine sacrifice. It's the brainwashing, the illusions, the confusion, the doubts, the uncertainty, the fears and the waiting for nothing to happen that causes the misery.

With Easyway we get rid of all the brainwashing, the fears, the doubts, the confusion and the uncertainty before we extinguish the final cigarette. When we extinguish that final cigarette, there's no feeling of sacrifice, no doom or gloom, just sheer elation because we know that we are already non-smokers, know that there is nothing to give up, know that we are already free, know that we've achieved what every smoker on the planet would love to achieve:

TO ESCAPE FROM THE NICOTINE PRISON

So that when we extinguish that final cigarette, we are not hoping or waiting to become non-smokers:

WE ARE ALREADY HAPPY NON-SMOKERS

In Chapter 4 I listed many common illusions that society generally still believes to be true even in this enlightened day. It is imperative that we remove all these illusions. However, to fully understand smoking, it is necessary to clarify another sinister aspect of the nicotine trap.

I've likened smoking to a lifetime of wearing tight shoes to get the pleasure of taking them off. Obviously it's far worse than that. It doesn't cost a fortune to wear tight shoes, you don't risk awful diseases and it's not a particularly filthy and disgusting pastime. Even so, we might occasionally wear tight shoes for reasons of necessity or vanity, but the biggest idiot on earth wouldn't wear them just to get the pleasure of removing them.

Wearing tight shoes has two other distinct advantages over smoking. When we are allowed to remove them, there is no little monster enticing us to put them on again. But the main advantage is: when you remove tight shoes your feet soon return to normal. You might have noticed that I have previously stated: when you light up, you partially relieve the empty, insecure feeling. Perhaps you have wondered why it isn't relieved completely.

It is because nicotine is an addictive drug and a powerful poison. Your body builds up an immunity to the poison which means it also builds up an immunity to the drug. The effect is that when you light a cigarette to relieve the empty, insecure feeling caused by the previous cigarette, you only partially relieve it.

So when you light a cigarette you don't even get back to feeling like a non-smoker again. You still feel less nervous or more relaxed than you did before you lit the cigarette and therefore your brain is still fooled into believing you got some genuine crutch or pleasure.

With a destructive pastime like smoking the natural tendency should be to smoke less and less. You don't need me to tell you that with drug addiction the tendency is to need more and more. The lower the drug drags you down, the more immune your body becomes to it, the more your brain craves for the illusory prop. This is an opportune moment to explain:

WHY CUTTING DOWN CANNOT WORK

17

WHY CUTTING DOWN CANNOT WORK

Terrible things happen when you try to cut down. First, you keep the little nicotine monster in your body alive, but more important, you keep the large monster in your brain craving cigarettes. Secondly, you spend your whole life clock-watching, wishing your life away waiting for your next fix. However, there are two worse things that happen when you try to cut down. When you indulge yourself cigarette after cigarette, at least you are partially relieving your withdrawal symptoms most of the time. When you cut down, in addition to the normal stresses and strains of life, you're actually causing yourself to feel nervous and insecure.

But the worst thing that happens is this: when you smoke cigarette after cigarette, you don't suffer the illusion of enjoying any of them. Even the lighting up becomes automatic. If you think about it, the so-called 'special' cigarettes are always the ones after a period of abstinence: the one after a meal, the first in the morning, the one after sex, the one after exercise and the one after a period of not being allowed to smoke. This is because all you actually enjoy when you light a cigarette is the ending of the aggravation of craving it, not the cigarette iself. Just like a hunger for food, the longer you suffer it, the more precious it becomes when you eventually relieve it. Cutting down doesn't turn smokers against smoking; on the contrary, it convinces them that the most precious thing in the world is the next cigarette.

Smokers make the mistake of believing that they smoke because they got into the habit of smoking and, in particular, that they got into the habit of smoking too many. We think that if we can restrict ourselves to smoking only five or ten a day, or just smoking those so-called 'special' cigarettes, our brains and bodies will get used to smoking at that level and we can happily maintain our smoking at that level or cut down further if we want to. If you have tried cutting down, you will know from experience that it just doesn't work. The reason it cannot work is because smoking isn't habit but drug addiction.

All smokers have this permanent nicotine itch inside their bodies. The natural tendency with an itch is to scratch it, and because smoking, far from curing the nicotine itch, actually causes it, the natural tendency for all smokers is to scratch it permanently or, in other words, to chain-smoke.

So why don't all smokers soon become chain-smokers? Because of the powerful forces on the other side of the tug-of-war which are telling us not to smoke. I used to think that my chain-smoking was a weakness. I thought: how can my friends limit their smoking to five or ten a day? I know I'm stronger-willed than they are.

It never occurred to me that some people are physically incapable of chain-smoking. You need strong lungs to chain-smoke. In the bad old days when smoking was regarded as a social pastime and 90 percent of adult males were hooked, the main reason that the other 10 percent didn't get hooked was because their lungs couldn't cope with the poison, or they hadn't got the will-power to go through the learning process. In those days we didn't have the benefit of filter-tips or low-tar tobaccos and the learning process was very difficult.

Many smokers can't afford to become heavy smokers and have to limit their intake according to their pocket. Others aren't allowed to smoke at work. Nowadays many smokers discipline themselves not to smoke in the bedroom, in a new car, in the company of non-smokers or whatever. Many youngsters will not smoke in the company of their parents and many parents will not smoke in the presence of their children or grand-children.

Although health is the main reason that smokers give for wanting to quit, the actual reason why so many mature smokers are attempting to quit nowadays is that smokers themselves regard it as anti-social. Even the illusion of the tough male or sophisticated lady has gone.

We don't particularly enjoy being smokers when we are young, but because we can cope with the physical side it doesn't appear to be a problem at that stage. However, because your body becomes immune to the drug, you always want more and more. Eventually you descend to the level of all drug addicts, where your body can no longer cope with the poisoning. Now you have not just one problem but two: at one and the same time you are smoking too much but can never get enough nicotine.

Even to hold it at the unacceptable level you are at, you would have to use will-power and discipline for the rest of your life. If you haven't got enough will-power to quit, no way will you have enough will-power to cut down. This is why cutting down cannot work. Cutting down usually follows a failed attempt to quit. Will-power runs out, and when it does the smokers are exhausted, miserable with self-despising and consequently end up smoking more than they did before they decided to quit.

Cutting down is closely associated with a group of smokers that heavy smokers tend to envy. Now is a good time to dispel another illusion:

THE MYTH OF THE HAPPY CASUAL SMOKER

18

THE MYTH OF THE HAPPY CASUAL SMOKER

It's not the chain-smoker coughing up his lungs that tempts us to experiment with those first cigarettes. We can see so clearly that they get no pleasure whatsoever from smoking and that it is smoking that is making their lives so miserable. What tempts us are the happy casual smokers. They have no smoker's cough, they look healthy and serene. It's quite obvious they are not addicts. Sometimes they'll take a cigarette out and not even bother to light it for several minutes. They are clearly in complete control.

It is this belief that it is possible to control your smoking that makes us put off the evil day when we try to quit. It is this same belief that other smokers are in control, enjoying their cigarettes, that makes us feel deprived and envious when we have quit.

They may be in control for the time being, but happy smokers they are not. I know this is difficult to believe, but there is no such person as a happy smoker, casual or otherwise. I could write a whole book on casual smoking. Unfortunately, I have many other aspects to cover and so must limit myself to one chapter.

In Chapter 5 I asked you to re-read the first few paragraphs. I would like you to re-read them again now. I would also remind you that the only reason any smoker lights a cigarette is to end the aggravation of craving it. Now, I realize that I might not have convinced you of this fact, but I promise you that before you have finished reading this book, I will. In the meantime, please trust me.

A five-a-day smoker scratches the itch for about an hour a day; the other 23 hours he suffers it. Because that empty, insecure feeling is identical to normal hunger and stress, the casual smoker doesn't relate it to smoking.

This is why casual smokers appear to enjoy it when they do eventually light up. Like wearing tight shoes, the longer you wear them the greater the relief when you eventually allow yourself to remove them. This also explains why younger, casual smokers are more hooked than older, heavier smokers. If you only smoke a few a day, the effect on your health and pocket are less than the heavy smoker's. At the same time the illusion of pleasure is greater. The overall effect is you have less reason to quit and a greater desire to continue. When we first start smoking, we don't even realize that we are in a prison, so why should we even want to escape from it? No way will you escape unless you want to. At least advanced addicts have a desire to escape and many succeed. The effect is that youngsters and casual smokers are more hooked than heavy smokers.

At the group clinics, when a casual smoker says something like, "I only smoke five a day", the heavy smokers stare with wonder at that smoker: "What are you doing here? I'd pay a thousand pounds if I could just smoke five a day."

The casual smoker's mere presence at the clinic proves my point. Casual smokers aren't happy smokers. In fact, some of the most pathetic people that attend our clinics are not the 60-a-day merchants, but casual smokers. I could give you a thousand examples. I'll restrict it to two.

The first was a young woman who attended my clinic in the days before I gave group sessions. She had been smoking just one cigarette a day for three months. I said, "I'm surprised you bother to consult me if you only smoke one a day." She started to cry and in between the tears managed to tell me her story:

"I was on 40 a day. I've got two beautiful children. They kept on at me – please stop smoking, we don't want you to die. I thought: 40 a day, surely it can't be too difficult to cut out one each day, and providing I keep doing that I must end up a non-smoker."

She finally got down to one a day but couldn't get rid of that final one. Her family believed that she had stopped completely. This is how she described her life:

"I'd get my husband off to work and my children off to school and then enjoy my cigarette. But if I smoked it, I'd have to go the rest of the day without one. So I'd say to myself: do the dishes first, then the dusting, then the ironing and so on."

Just before her children came home from school she would smoke that cigarette. Now, in her rational mind she was just one cigarette away from being a non-smoker. But what was the true position? She wasn't getting off smoking – on the contrary, now her whole life was being dominated by that one cigarette. Dangling this carrot all day, every day under her nose, desperately hoping that, provided she could hang out long enough, eventually she would lose the desire to smoke. But was that one cigarette less precious? Of course not. All she did was ingrain into her mind that the most precious thing on earth is a cigarette and that she couldn't enjoy life without one. If ever you've been through a bout of cutting down, the circumstances might be different, but I'm sure you found the same result.

The second example was at the time that I was doing group clinics and I was so busy that I was no longer able to do individual sessions. A lady rang up pleading for an individual session and began to cry when I explained that it had to be part of a group session or not at all. I'm a sucker for tears and agreed to an individual session.

You would be forgiven for believing that this lady was a weak person, using her feminine wiles to manipulate a gullible male. You would be wrong. She turned out to be one of the strongest characters I have ever met, a famous barrister at the peak of her profession. This is what she told me:

"I hated smoking as a youngster. Both of my parents were heavy smokers and both eventually died of lung cancer. I can't explain why I was so stupid as to try one but I did about 12 years ago. Because I had this great fear that I would get lung cancer, I've never smoked more than two cigarettes a day and I never smoke less than two."

It's very difficult to persuade heavy smokers that there is no such thing as a happy smoker, casual or otherwise. This is because we all start off as casual smokers. We therefore know that it is possible to be in that blissful state. Was it so blissful? Fortunately, most of us can remember how unpleasant those first experimental cigarettes were. Now look back at the stage when you'd learned to cope with the filth but were still a casual smoker. Did those cigarettes really taste so good? Can you remember all those wonderful cigarettes you smoked? Or was it only when you couldn't smoke that those cigarettes appeared to be so precious?

The other reason we believe there are happy casual smokers in complete control is that we meet them every day and they tell us they can take them or leave them. Think of Chapter 5 again. Do you really believe anyone who could take them or leave them would actually take them? Another fact you need to get clearly in your mind is:

ALL SMOKERS ARE LIARS

I don't mean that they are basically dishonest people. In all other respects they might be honest, but about their smoking they lie. It's not their fault; they have to and the worst part is that they lie to themselves.

Do you think the lady barrister broke down in tears in front of her friends and colleagues and told them how stupid she was to have started smoking after both her parents had died from lung cancer, or telling them of the misery of those twelve years terrified that she too would contract the disease and having to discipline herself to only be allowed to scratch that itch just twice a day? That lady was too intelligent to deceive herself. If asked she would simply say: "I only need two a day." She might not have deliberately lied to her acquaintances, but I wonder how many of them envied her and misquoted her:

SHE QUITE HAPPILY SMOKES JUST TWO A DAY

Because all smokers instinctively feel stupid, we have to pretend that we do get some pleasure or crutch in order to retain some semblance of self-respect in our own eyes and in the eyes of others. If only all smokers would be completely honest and declare their hatred of smoking, the whole nightmare would rapidly disintegrate. It's only the belief that millions of smokers do enjoy it that gets us hooked in the first place, keeps us hooked and gets us hooked again if we do manage to escape for a while.

If you have followed the instructions, you will already have learned that most cigarettes are smoked subconsciously. The reason for this is that if you had to smoke every cigarette consciously, like the one I asked you to smoke in Chapter 4, and had to be aware of the foul effects; if you had to say to yourself: "This might just be the one to trigger off cancer in my lungs and I'm going to spend a small fortune in my lifetime of filth and slavery", then even the illusion of pleasure goes. The fear of quitting makes us block our minds to the evils of smoking, but even when we try to do that we still feel stupid. If we had to face up to it every time we lit up, it would be intolerable.

We've all heard a casual smoker say something like: "Oh, it doesn't bother me. I can go all week without a cigarette." Why do all smokers brag about how little they smoke? When I was addicted to golf, I would brag about how often I played. I wasn't ashamed of it and I wanted to play more. If I said to you: "I can go all week without carrots", on the surface I'm telling you that I have no problem with carrots. If I genuinely have no problem with carrots, why would I bother to make a statement like that? Smokers that brag about going long periods without cigarettes are entitled to brag, because they have exercised will-power and discipline and feel proud of themselves. They've proved to themselves that they are in control. If they are genuinely in control, why do they have to smoke one after that week of abstinence?

If there is a genuine crutch or pleasure from smoking, why would anyone want to deprive themselves of that pleasure for a whole week? If there is no genuine pleasure, why would they need to smoke one at the end of the week?

Let's briefly examine the main groups of casual smoker. There are the ones that dabble and either through luck or fear never get hooked. That's the type that will have one cigarette or cigar at Christmas and never smoke during the rest of the year. Remember, non-smokers are also subjected to the lifetime's brainwashing, and many of them feel that they are missing out. They don't enjoy that cigarette; in fact it tastes foul. In order to suffer the illusion of enjoyment, you have to become immune to the foul effect and to do that you have to smoke regularly. Don't envy them. If that cigarette tasted gorgeous, would you really want to have to wait a whole year for it? The other reason you shouldn't envy them is that even though they might manage to restrict their smoking for years, sooner or later the vast majority of them become hooked completely.

The second type of casual smoker is one that is hooked, but is only at the beginning of the slide down. Some, like me, go sliding down in a matter of a few months. With most smokers it is a matter of a few years.

The third type is very rare. The lady barrister is a classic example of smokers who exercise immense will-power and remain casual smokers for years. They are effectively more hooked and more miserable than any other type. I envy them their will-power and pity them for the misery it causes them.

The fourth type is the heavy smoker who is cutting down after a failed attempt to quit. Although we might feel proud of ourselves at the outset, like the lady who tried to cut out one cigarette a day, eventually we end up smoking more than previously. But, of course, it is during the period that we are successful that we find the need to tell other smokers how little we smoke. Another type that other smokers tend to envy, who are not necessarily casual smokers, are the stoppers and starters. They are so lucky and in complete control. They can happily smoke for six months, then happily quit for six months.

BULLSHIT!

If they are genuinely happy smoking for six months, why don't they go on happily smoking for the rest of their lives? If they can happily quit for six months, why don't they remain happy non-smokers for the rest of their lives? We think they get the best of all worlds: when they want to be smokers they smoke and when they want to be non-smokers they don't smoke.

The reason they decide to quit is exactly the same reason you and I decide to quit: because we don't like being smokers. When they do quit, they feel deprived and miserable and wish they could smoke again. Eventually their will-power runs out and they start smoking again. Do they say: "I started again because I'm a weak-willed jellyfish that failed to quit"? Of course not. They have to try to retain some self-respect. The truth is that they get the worst of all worlds. When they are smokers, they wish they were non-smokers and when they are non-smokers, they wish they were smokers.

Isn't this true of our whole smoking lives? When we are allowed to smoke, we wish we didn't have to. It's only when we aren't allowed to smoke that cigarettes appear so precious.

One other classification of casual smoking is the worst of all: the secret smoker. You are ashamed to tell your family and friends that you failed to quit. You deceive and deliberately avoid the presence of the people you most love and the people whose company you most enjoy.

You sneak off to the garage or wherever. You light the cigarette, it tastes foul. You've now reached rock bottom. You've lost all semblance of self-respect. You think: "Why am I doing this? What is the power that this evil holds over me?" You might still be deceiving other people, but you can no longer deceive yourself. You know:

YOU ARE A PATHETIC DRUG ADDICT!

With the brainwashed mind of the smoker, it's easy to be fooled into believing some casual smokers are in control and happy to be smokers. But once you understand the nicotine trap, it's easy to see them in their true light. The self-deceit becomes so obvious. The most powerful influence to make you happy to be a non-smoker is to observe other smokers. A good time to observe casual smokers is at social occasions:

"I only smoke five a day."
"But you've smoked three while I've been talking to you."
"Oh, parties are different."

Many casual smokers will almost chain-smoke at social events. Watch after they extinguish one cigarette how quickly they begin to get restless. I call it the smoker's twitch. Notice how they look around hoping someone else will light up. Notice how quickly they offer the cigarettes around if nobody else does. Watch the first few puffs. You can almost feel their sense of relief. Notice from that point on they don't even seem to be aware that they are smoking. Notice how quickly the cigarette seems to burn. Watch the filth they are breathing into their lungs. Imagine the nicotine leaving their body and how quickly the twitching starts again. See that lifelong chain as it really is, unless of course:

YOU ARE LUCKY ENOUGH TO BREAK IT!

Incidentally, when you observe other smokers, do so unobtrusively. You might be tempted to point out that you see through their façade, thinking it will help them to quit. Avoid the temptation, you will only succeed in embarrassing them and making yourself unpopular. Remember, it is only fear that keeps people smoking. To attempt to force a smoker to quit who is not ready to quit is like trying to force someone who suffers from claustrophobia into a crowded elevator. They will kill you to avoid it.

While we are on the subject, soon you will experience the many joys of being free, and one of those is to help your smoking friends and relatives to share your joy. Your natural instinct will be to lecture them. Don't try, play it softly, softly. If the subject comes up, don't even attempt to explain the mysteries of the little monster and the big monster. Just keep telling them how lovely it is to be free. This will not only arouse their curiosity, but also help to remove their fear. Soon they will approach you with an open and receptive mind. Then you will have the pleasure of helping them to escape. However, we must first ensure that you escape. Let's consider:

EXACTLY WHAT YOU ARE TRYING TO ACHIEVE?

19

WHAT ARE YOU TRYING TO ACHIEVE?

That's obvious: to stop smoking. No, that's what smokers who use the 'will-power' method do, or to put it another way: they try never to smoke again. Simply expressing it that way makes it appear like a lifetime's task.

What is the real difference between a smoker and a non-smoker? Again the answer is obvious: a smoker smokes and a non-smoker doesn't. No, that is simply the result of the difference. The real difference is that a smoker has a need or desire to smoke whereas a non-smoker has no need or desire to smoke.

THAT IS WHAT WE MUST ACHIEVE

You don't want to become one of these complaining stoppers who spend the rest of their lives craving the occasional cigarette, feeling deprived and having to resist temptation. You've no doubt heard the expression frequently used by smokers who tried to quit smoking using the 'will-power' method: "I feel like a smoker who isn't allowed to smoke." You don't need to be one of them. In Chapter 13 I said smoking is negative. If your objective is not to do something for the rest of your life, how can you be sure that you've succeeded until you've lived the rest of your life? You might conclude you can never be truly free until you've lived the rest of your life. I promise you that you can.

I assume that you have no desire to inject heroin into a vein. Do you spend the rest of your life worrying about not being allowed to do it? Of course not, because you have no desire to do it. You might argue, "But I've never been a heroin addict." So what? Neither have I. I have been a nicotine addict, but I have no more desire to smoke than I have to inject myself with heroin.

So, once we've removed the desire to smoke, and taken precautions to ensure that the desire never returns, we are already free. What we are trying to achieve is a frame of mind. Now, you might be having a good day or a bad day. Either way it doesn't occur to you to inject yourself with heroin; you just accept it and enjoy it or cope with it.

However, if it did occur to you to inject yourself with heroin, whether it be a good day or a bad day, you wouldn't do it. What we are going to do is to get you into a certain frame of mind: when you have extinguished that final cigarette, when it occurs to you to light a cigarette, whether it be a good day or a bad day, instead of feeling the need to light one or feeling miserable because you're not allowed to light one, you think:

ISN'T IT GREAT! I DON'T NEED ONE! I'M A NON-SMOKER!

This begs the question:

WHEN DO YOU BECOME A NON-SMOKER?

It is essential that you think about this question before continuing, because it is one of the keys to success. Typical answers are:

• When I stop thinking about it.
• When I can enjoy a social occasion.
• When I can answer the phone.

A common answer is "You never do; once a smoker always a smoker, you're just a smoker who can't smoke." With all these answers you are waiting for something to happen. How long will you have to wait? I once survived six months on the 'will-power' method. It never happened. It is this waiting and uncertainty that make quitting so difficult.

Get it clear in your mind:

YOU BECOME A NON-SMOKER THE MOMENT YOU EXTINGUISH YOUR FINAL CIGARETTE!

Unless you are certain, you will only be hoping that it's your final cigarette and the chances are you'll wait in vain.

But how can you possibly be certain that it will be your final cigarette?

BY REMOVING THE UNCERTAINTY FIRST!

The causes of the uncertainty are all the illusions listed in Chapter 4, the belief that we get some genuine pleasure or crutch from smoking, that it's difficult to quit and that, even if we succeed, life will never be as enjoyable again.

At my clinics, when I am only halfway through the session a smoker might say: "You needn't say another word, Allen. I see it so clearly. I know I'll never smoke again!"

This usually happens after I've explained the concept that smoking is like wearing tight shoes. Usually those smokers are people like myself who were almost at the bottom of the nicotine pit and could not accept the many misconceptions perpetuated by society. Perhaps you are one of these people. If so, I must ask you to be tolerant with me. I have already dealt at length with the subject. However, most smokers find it difficult to accept the concept immediately and in order to remove uncertainty it is absolutely necessary for you to know that:

THERE ARE NO ADVANTAGES WHATSOEVER IN BEING A SMOKER

Smoking is simply a version of nicotine addiction. What do you think the 21st century's version will be? Is your money on nicotine gum or patches? Do you find the suggestion far-fetched? Unless you open your mind and help me to educate the rest of society about the true facts of nicotine addiction, it could well be one of those. We've already had hundreds of people visit our clinics who have actually quit smoking and seek our help because they are hooked on nicotine gum.

Perhaps your money is on the latest fad: nasal sprays containing nicotine. Perhaps you find that even more far-fetched. Before you dismiss the suggestion as outrageous, let's examine for a moment the form of nicotine addiction adopted in previous centuries:

SNUFF-TAKING

20

SNUFF-TAKING

In case you are not aware, snuff is simply dried tobacco. The 'habit' had many similarities to smoking. It was considered to be a very sociable pastime. Unfortunately, the most prominent memory that I have of my maternal grand-mother is of the brown dew-drop that hung permanently from her nose. How could such a disgusting 'habit' possibly be regarded as sociable?

For years smoking was widely accepted as a sociable 'habit'. How could you possibly describe a pastime that involves polluting the atmosphere with obnoxious and toxic fumes as sociable? It's about as sociable as an emission of wind in an elevator.

Why was either filthy, disgusting pastime regarded as sociable? Because when you get hooked on any drug you feel stupid. If you can find someone equally stupid, you don't feel quite so bad. If you can find a whole group of people equally stupid, you might even begin to think: "I can't be stupid, there must be something in it, otherwise all these other intelligent people wouldn't be doing it." All drug addicts tend to group together. A client once told me:

"I was at a party. I spent the entire evening talking to this man that I found quite objectionable. It wasn't until the next day that it dawned on me: he was the only other smoker there; he could have been Dracula and it wouldn't have made the slightest difference."

Nowadays in restaurants, if you invite a lone smoker to smoke, they'll say: "I never smoke at a meal when non-smokers are present." That is not because they are particularly considerate, but because they feel unsociable, stupid and uncomfortable smoking in the presence of non-smokers. However, if you are the lone non-smoker, those same considerate people will be puffing away, not just after the meal, but between courses and even during courses. Both snuff-taking and smoking are filthy, disgusting pastimes and their participants tried to cover up the fact by introducing attractive accessories. With snuff-taking it was the silver snuff-box. With smoking it was the gold and silver cigarette cases, the expensive lighters. Have you noticed how rarely you see one of those cigarette cases nowadays? Even the expensive lighters have gone out of fashion. All smokers seem to use the cheap throwaways. That's because since smoking became unsociable even the illusion of pleasure has gone. All smokers are hoping to quit soon. Even when they get one of those expensive lighters as a present, they are saying: "That's wonderful, I'll treasure it all my life." But they are thinking: "Oh, no! Why didn't you ask me first? I'm going to quit!"

Just like smokers, snuff-takers would come out with the same irrational arguments to justify their stupidity:

"It clears my head."
"You mean it actually blows your brains out?"
"No, don't be stupid, I mean it makes me sneeze!"
"One of us is being stupid but I'm not convinced it's me. Why do you need to sneeze?"
"I told you, to clear my head."
"But if you didn't sniff the filth up your nose you wouldn't have to clear your head. In any case, if you want to sneeze, try pepper. It's much more effective, cheaper and less harmful."
"Oh, you are just trying to be awkward."

That is exactly what I'm trying not to be. Do you think heroin addicts inject themselves because they like injections? Of course not. They do it to get the heroin. Do you think cocaine addicts sniff because they enjoy sniffing? Of course not. They do it because they are addicted to cocaine. Do you really believe snuff-takers sniffed snuff because they enjoyed sniffing? If so, why not sniff pepper? Of course not. They did it for one reason and one reason alone, they were addicted to the most powerful drug known to mankind. They did it because:

THEY WERE ADDICTED TO NICOTINE!

If you can see clearly that people wouldn't be stupid enough to breathe dried tobacco up their noses for any other reason than that they were addicted to nicotine, you should be able to see with equal clarity that the only reason smokers spend a fortune to place poisonous sticks in their mouths, set light to them and actually breathe the filth into their lungs, is because:

THEY ARE ADDICTED TO NICOTINE!

We believe there is some inherent pleasure or comfort in breathing fumes into our lungs and that the health, the money, the nicotine addiction are just annoying side-effects to interfere with that pleasure. If only there were a safe cigarette. The tobacco companies have spent a fortune searching for a safe cigarette. Have you tried herbal cigarettes? If you have you will know that, just like normal cigarettes, they taste awful. However, unlike normal cigarettes, no matter how long you persevere with them, you will never suffer the illusion of enjoying them:

BECAUSE THEY DON'T CONTAIN NICOTINE

If you haven't now got that clearly into your mind, you need to go back to page one. Don't feel disappointed if you have to do that. Remember, you've been subjected to a lifetime's brainwashing. You might find it difficult to reverse it immediately. But it is essential that you do. How do I know that I am right, that what I'm telling you is the truth? As Sherlock Holmes says:

"Once you have eliminated the impossible, whatever remains, however improbable, must be the answer."

With drug addiction, once you understand it, the only remaining possibility isn't improbable, it is so obvious that you wonder how all of the people could have been fooled for so long. I once appeared on national TV with an eminent physician who stated: "Nicotine is a wonderful drug". This man actually purports to be an expert on helping smokers to quit. Naturally, he advocates NRT. An equally eminent physician also stated on national TV:

"It is possible that some heavy smokers may be so dependent on nicotine that, if they quit smoking, they will have to use a nicotine replacement permanently."

When so-called experts make such statements, is it surprising smokers find it so difficult to quit? The medical experts themselves seem to assist the tobacco industry by emphasizing that the main problem is not nicotine addiction itself, but smoking tobacco and inhaling the tars. It doesn't seem to occur to them that the only reason people smoke is because they are addicted to nicotine, and that if you can help them get free from nicotine addiction, they'll have no need to smoke tobacco or any other obnoxious fumes.

The point I wish to make is that it would be easy to draw the conclusion that, provided you don't smoke tobacco, dependence on – or addiction to – nicotine is not a particularly harmful pastime and might even be quite pleasant.

Perhaps the two eminent doctors drew their conclusions because thousands of ex-smokers are hooked on nicotine gum. Hundreds of nicotine gum addicts have attended our clinics and many were still actually smoking. I have the greatest respect for doctors and I am aware that they are far more expert than I on the harm smoking causes to the human body. Unfortunately, they generally have no idea of how to help smokers quit.

We need to be aware that doctors like to prescribe pills. NRT sounds logical and I will explain later why it's about as logical as saying to a person that smokes heroin: "Don't smoke heroin, smoking is dangerous, just inject it straight into your vein."

I'm grateful that the second eminent physician only suggested that it might be possible that some heavy ex-smokers would have to use nicotine replacement for the rest of their lives. Can you imagine the effect such a statement would have on a heavy smoker who already suspected that he was hooked for life?

I've often been accused by the established medical profession of being unscientific and I find it incredible that a qualified doctor would make such a statement without being certain. I'm suspicious of people, no matter how eminent they might be, who make suggestions that contradict the known facts. I'm even more suspicious of people who make categoric statements and are then proved to be wrong. My instructions will be completely categoric. During the 15 years that I and my colleagues have been helping smokers to escape from the nicotine prison, not a single person, so-called expert or otherwise, has been able to contradict my statements, either with the use of facts or logical scientific argument.

I have been accused of making unkind comments against the medical profession. Let me make it quite clear. I have the greatest respect for the medical profession. My youngest son is a qualified doctor and I couldn't be more proud. My greatest advocates are from the more open-minded members of the medical profession. We not only have more smokers seek the help of our clinics from the medical profession, but more clients are recommended to us by the medical profession than by any other. If I have been critical of the medical profession, the example of one of my failures will explain why:

"I followed your instructions to the letter. I even used nicotine gum and avoided smoking situations."
"But my instructions were not to use NRT and not to avoid smoking situations."
"I know but my doctor said it would make it easier."

I'm sure you see my problem. I've stated that Easyway will enable all smokers to find it easy to quit provided they follow all the instructions. In the example that I have given, the smoker clearly did not follow two of the instructions. So why do I describe her as my failure?

At our clinics we give a money-back guarantee. On the basis of that guarantee our worldwide success rate is in excess of 90 percent. Now, I don't need to have discovered an easy way to stop smoking in order to achieve a success rate of 100 percent. Keen gardeners will know the havoc created by slugs and that anyone who discovered a genuine solution to the problem would soon become a millionaire. A gardening expert once informed me that he responded to the following advert: "SLUG

KILLER. GUARANTEED WORKS EVERY TIME." He figured: "For the amount they're asking, what have I got to lose?" A month later a parcel arrived containing two blocks of wood and a set of simple instructions: "Place the slug on one block and bring the other block down on it with sufficient force to crush it."

Did the advertisers lie? No. Was the man cheated? Of course he was. Did the advertiser become a millionaire? I doubt it very much. They might have cheated some people, but once the confidence trick was discovered, future adverts were refused.

I could give a money-back guarantee that would enable all smokers to find it easy to quit provided they followed all the instructions. I would only need two instructions:

- Extinguish your last cigarette and never light another.
- For the rest of your life, whenever you think about smoking, think: "Isn't it wonderful, I'm a non-smoker."

If you just followed those instructions, you would actually find it easy to quit. How many smokers would actually succeed? I doubt whether it would be more than one in a thousand. But if you failed, it would be because you failed to followed one of those instructions. I'd claim that it was your fault. Would I have cheated you? Of course. Would I have been invited to speak at The World Conference on Health and Tobacco? No way! Would I have been described as a guru, a genius or a saint? No. I would have been described as what I would have actually been: a confidence trickster.

We don't renege on our guarantee because a smoker doesn't follow all the instructions. Our clients don't seek our help to waste our time or their own, and we take it on faith that they genuinely want to quit. Our function is not just to give a set of instructions to be followed regardless and then blame the smoker for failing to follow them. Our expertise is to enable each and every individual smoker to understand why they need to follow those instructions, to understand that not only have they been brainwashed in the past, but that the brainwashing and misinformation will continue in the future. It would have been easy to blame the failure on that lady because she relied on her doctor's advice. To do so wouldn't have done her any good and it certainly wouldn't have done me any good. Perhaps she wasn't the brightest person in the world, perhaps she had a bad day. It's immaterial. It was my function to enable her to so understand Easyway that even when an intelligent, altruistic, qualified physician contradicted the advice I was giving, she would ignore that contradiction and follow my advice. In the example that I have given, for whatever reason, I failed to achieve my object. It was my failure not hers.

At our clinics we have even refunded our fee to smokers who, although they haven't smoked, are still struggling. Our guarantee is to enable them to be happy non-smokers and unless we achieve that, we don't argue, there is no inquisition, we simply trust the smoker. Some people say that's an incredibly naive view from a chartered accountant. Is it? Imagine you were imprisoned for years and someone helped you to escape, would you cheat them?

I doubt it. I've helped to cure over 25,000 smokers personally. I know of only one case when a smoker tried to cheat me. He wrote me a very aggressive letter, claiming that the method hadn't worked and he wanted a refund. Amazingly, I got repeated recommendations from this person. One of them told me that the man had never smoked since he'd left the clinic. I said: "But he claimed a refund." He said: "I know, but he was going through a very bad time financially and has asked me to ask you to accept the money back and to forgive him."

You are in exactly the same position as smokers that attend our clinics. You will also be subjected to immense brainwashing for the rest of your life. You will also be given advice that might appear to be perfectly logical and yet contradict Easyway. It's no good you just accepting my instructions parrot fashion. You need to understand that, no matter how eminent or qualified that expert might be, no matter how many equally qualified so-called experts support his views, Easyway is the true map, not only to escape from the maze but to ensure that your escape is permanent.

Let's make it absolutely clear now. This book is entitled *The Easy Way to Stop Smoking*. It should be entitled:

THE EASY WAY TO BE FREE FROM NICOTINE ADDICTION

The only way to be free from smoking is to be free from nicotine addiction. All nicotine addiction. Whether it be nicotine gum, patches or nasal sprays, whether you chew tobacco or sniff snuff, it's equivalent to banging your head against a wall to make it nice to quit.

If you have fully understood what I have written so far you will know that when I use the word cigarettes, I might just as well have said cigars or a pipe. Part of the trap is always to switch to some other form of nicotine intake in order to postpone the evil day, and another part is to claim that cigars/pipes are not as dangerous as smoking cigarettes. More panic thinking. It might be more dangerous to take arsenic than strychnine. It is obviously more dangerous to fall from the third floor than the second. But would an intelligent individual use these as rational arguments for doing either?

Obviously not. Once you realize that it is only the fear and panic caused by drug addiction that makes us come out with such ridiculous statements, and more important, once you can see clearly that the only reason we continue to smoke is to try to get back to that blissful state we had permanently before we became addicted to nicotine, then we can increase the certainty by:

REVERSING THE BRAINWASHING

21

REVERSING THE BRAINWASHING

In order to be certain it is essential to reverse all of the brainwashing. Please refer back to the list of illusions and misconceptions at the beginning of Chapter 4. Please note that we have already dispelled the first 8.

Now let's remove Nos 9 to 12. How can the same cigarette assist opposites like boredom and concentration or relaxing and stressful situations? Obviously it can't. It is just a cunning illusion. Not only doesn't it help any of these situations, it actually makes them worse.

How is the illusion created? Because the little nicotine monster is a permanent itch. If the smoker has something to occupy his mind which isn't stressful, he isn't even aware of it. However, in a bored or relaxed state, he has nothing to take his mind off it, and scratches the itch by lighting up. Just think about it: boredom is a frame of mind. What is so mind-absorbing about smoking a cigarette? In fact, can you visualize a more boring pastime than someone like me chain-smoking cigarette after cigarette? We assume it relieves boredom because that is one of the occasions when we feel the need to scratch the itch. In fact, smoking is a strong contributor to boredom for two powerful reasons. First, as the gunging-up process imperceptibly makes us feel more and more lethargic, we no longer have the energy to continue pastimes that would occupy our minds. Secondly, as our illusory dependence on the drug grows, the panic feeling that the man on the yacht experienced when he discovered that he'd forgotten his cigarettes tends to take a greater hold over us. We either consciously or subconsciously avoid situations in which we aren't allowed to smoke.

In hindsight I believe that golf became my pet sport because it was the only active sport that I could play and smoke at the same time. My non-smoking friends were still playing soccer, tennis and squash years after I gave them up.

Why does smoking appear to aid concentration? Because any distraction will impede concentration. The little monster creates a permanent distraction. The telephone rings. You don't even have to think about it. You automatically light a cigarette. You are actually better able to concentrate than a moment before, because you have partially relieved the distraction, but because you have only partially relieved it, you are still less able to concentrate than you will be once the little monster has died.

Smoking also impedes concentration in a much more serious way. As a smoker, you increasingly replace oxygen with carbon monoxide and nutrients with poisons. The essential oxygen and nutrients are supplied by your blood. Smoking not only coagulates your blood but gunges up your arteries, veins and capillaries. Which organ of your body most relies on an efficient supply of blood? At the clinics this question is often greeted with silly grins on the men's faces. Although smoking does have a substantial debilitating effect on a husband's capacity to fulfil his marital responsibilities, the actual organ I refer to is the brain.

Chain-smoking is a nightmare. Every time you really need a cigarette you are already smoking one. The telephone would ring and I would extinguish the cigarette I was smoking in order to get the crutch of lighting another one. Occasionally I would find that I had two going at the same time. That's when you begin to suspect that the cigarette is doing absolutely nothing for you.

For most smokers the best cigarette is the one after a meal. But why should the same cigarette out of the same packet taste different after a meal? Of course it doesn't. We've already established that if a smoker can't get their own brand, they'll smoke old rope rather than nothing. Even the expression 'after a meal' is a fallacy. Most smokers smoke between courses and some will smoke during courses.

Cigarettes only appear to taste better after meals because a meal is a genuinely pleasant experience, particularly the evening meal when our work for the day is over and we can sit down and relax. The pleasure is increased when the meal is at a restaurant with friends. This is because we've removed two other possible causes of aggravation: we have pleasant company and aren't bored, and we're being waited on. We remove two other aggravations: our hunger and our thirst. When we've done all these things we should be completely relaxed and on a high. Non-smokers will be. But smokers won't be able to relax until they've satisfied the nicotine monster.

Smoking doesn't improve meals. On the contrary it ruins your taste-buds and your sense of smell. One of the great joys of being free is to be able to enjoy the taste and smell of food again, and to be able to sit there truly enjoying the meal rather than wishing everyone would hurry up and finish their meal so that you can scratch the itch.

We think smoking helps to relax us at parties. We stand there drink in one hand, cigarette in the other. We don't want to dance, partly because we have no energy, but mainly because it means we will have to extinguish our cigarette. Some smokers are so hooked they can't even do that. They smooch round a crowded dance floor with a lighted cigarette. How pathetic! I know just how pathetic – I used to be one of them.

It's not that smokers enjoy smoking after meals or at parties, it's just that they are in a panic without them. Meals and parties are genuinely enjoyable and exciting occasions for non-smokers. The reason why those cigarettes appear to be so special is that they make the difference between being relaxed and utterly miserable. Always remember: the cigarette itself never tastes any different. It is always poisonous, foul and unpleasant. It's the occasion when you partially relieve the itch that makes some cigarettes appear to be more precious than others. The cigarette doesn't relieve this feeling of anxiety. On the contrary, it is the cause of it. Non-smokers don't suffer from that anxious feeling – neither did you before you got hooked and, although you might find it difficult to believe, you won't suffer from it again once we've killed both monsters.

Why does smoking appear to relieve stress? Let's use an example: let's imagine that you and I are identical twins. The only difference between us is that you are addicted to nicotine and I am not. Tomorrow we both have a dental appointment that will cause us to wake up feeling somewhat stressed. However, you will feel more stressed than I because you will have gone all night without nicotine. You won't blame that extra stress on the fact that you are a smoker, because smokers believe that smoking helps to relieve stress, not cause it. In your mind it will all be blamed on the visit to the dentist.

You will light a cigarette and immediately feel less stressed than a moment before, thereby reinforcing your belief that cigarettes help to relieve stress. But will you now be completely happy? Will you be thinking: "Who cares about going to the dentist?" Of course you won't. If smoking genuinely relieved stress, smokers' lives would be all honey and roses and you wouldn't even be reading this book.

Even while you are smoking that cigarette you will still feel more stressed than me. You haven't solved the visit to the dentist, you still have to go. All you have done is partially relieve the stress caused by the little monster. When you are at the dentist you will be even worse off because you won't be allowed to even partially relieve the aggravation. This is another evil about smoking that never seems to occur to us: at some of the most stressful periods in our lives, we aren't even allowed to partially relieve our withdrawal symptoms.

When we leave the dentist I will have a big smile on my face because I will be completely stress-free. You won't feel completely stress-free until you can light up and feed the monster. Even then you won't be completely free. You've forgotten what it is to feel completely relaxed. That's another joy that you can look forward to.

While we're on the subject of stress, let's explode the next myth:

I SMOKE BECAUSE I SUFFER WITH MY NERVES

22

I SMOKE BECAUSE I SUFFER
WITH MY NERVES

No. It's the other way around – you suffer with your nerves because you smoke. I was halfway through one of my early group clinics. It was a stifling July day so I left the door open. Suddenly it slammed and one elderly client jumped two feet in the air and said: "You can see the state of my nerves. How will I survive without smoking?"

There were sympathetic nods from the rest of the group. I could well understand their view. When I was a boy, in sports like snooker, darts or pool all the top players were heavy smokers. It seemed obvious that smoking helped them to control their nerves. I can remember watching 'Hurricane' Higgins, the world snooker champion. His face had a permanent twitch. He couldn't keep still. When he lit up he would almost swallow the cigarette. You could see his cheeks trying to extract the nicotine. Because from birth I had been brainwashed to believe that smoking helped to relax the nerves, the sight of 'Hurricane' Higgins lighting up only served to reinforce that brainwashing. It never occurred to me that the nervousness was being increased by the little monster rather than relieved by it. It's amazing how obvious it becomes when you stop looking at smoking through rose-coloured spectacles. Over the next two decades two players dominated the world of snooker: Steve Davis and Stephen Hendry, both non-smokers. They certainly helped to explode the myth that smoking helps to relax the nerves.

I can remember how I would go berserk when one of my children did something wrong. My reaction was out of all proportion to the misdemeanour. I really believed that I had a serious flaw in my character and that smoking helped to relax me. It wasn't until I quit that I realized that the flaw was the little nicotine monster.

A few years ago there was a radio phone-in to gauge reaction to a threat by the adoption authorities to forbid smokers from adopting children. A man rang up irate: "It is sheer nonsense. I remember when we were children, if we had some contentious item to raise with our mother, we would wait until she lit a cigarette. It was so obvious that she was more relaxed when she was smoking."

That's what we've all been brain-washed to believe. It didn't occur to the man to question why she was so unrelaxed when she wasn't smoking, or why even at times like after meals, when non-smokers are totally relaxed, smokers cannot relax without smoking.

Check it out for yourself. The next time you are in a supermarket and see a young housewife screaming at a child out of all proportion to the crime it has committed, notice the first thing she'll do when she gets outside will be to light a cigarette. You even see people smoking while riding a bicycle or scooter. Do you really believe that they can possibly be enjoying that cigarette?

We've now cleared up the first 13 of the 22 illusions listed in Chapter 4. Now let's deal with No.14:

ARE SMOKERS STUPID?

The simple answer is 'no', unless the smoker believes that they aren't stupid, in which case the answer is 'yes'. This statement might appear to be contradictory. It might also appear to be confusing. Allow me to elaborate.

On one of my failed attempts to quit when using the 'will-power' method, I listed on a piece of paper as many arguments against smoking as I could think of. It came to over 30. The idea is that every time you have the slightest temptation to smoke, you take out your list and before you've got through the first five items you resist the temptation.

If any smoker were to list all the disadvantages of smoking on one side and all the advantages on the other, then allocate points out of ten to each item and add up the totals, the answer would be – a dozen times over –

IT IS STUPID TO SMOKE!

This is why all smokers hate the thought of their children smoking and why all smokers instinctively feel stupid. You may feel stupid, but remember: you didn't make a conscious decision to become a smoker; on the contrary, you were lured into an ingenious trap.

Perhaps you are tempted to try the method I described above. After all, it sounds quite logical. Please don't waste your time. If you have already experimented with a similar method, you will already have discovered that it doesn't work. Why doesn't it work? Because in spite of your list, and for the reasons I have already explained, your brain continues to crave cigarettes and you feel increasingly deprived and miserable. Eventually your resistance runs out until you reach the stage when the next time you are tempted, you still take out your list but instead of reading it you tear it up into little pieces.

You see, nothing changed because you actually listed all the stupidities of being a smoker. All you were doing was confirming what you had known all your life:

SMOKING IS STUPID

All your list did was prevent you from doing what the other side of your brain desperately wanted you to do: light a cigarette. In fact, it didn't prevent you – it simply prolonged the agony. We all know that smoking is stupid, but that doesn't necessarily mean that smokers are stupid.

Did you ever attempt to solve Rubik's cube? I love such puzzles and pride myself on my ability to solve them. I spent two weeks trying to solve Rubik's cube. The only firm conclusion that I came to was:

"If I had to spend the rest of my life in prison until I had solved Rubik's cube, then I would have spent the rest of my life in prison."

Even when someone gave me a leaflet explaining how to solve Rubik's cube, it took me another two weeks to solve it. However, like all puzzles, no matter how ingenious they are, once you know the answer it's easy.

Is the nicotine trap more ingenious than Rubik's cube? I leave you to be the judge of that. I don't know how many people have solved Rubik's cube unaided. I don't even know whether Rubik himself could solve the problem. Obviously someone did, otherwise I'd never have known how to do it. All I do know is that out of the millions of smokers that have lived and died, I was the first to solve the mystery of quitting smoking.

All my smoking life I despised myself, first for being stupid enough to fall into the trap and secondly for not having the sense or will-power to quit. Smoking is the most sinister, ingenious trap that man and nature have combined to lay, not only because of how cleverly it traps its victims, but also the cunning way it keeps them trapped for life.

Smoking is stupid but smokers aren't. You are reading this book because you know smoking is stupid. Earlier I related the incident of a client who resented the fact that he couldn't quit of his own will-power and had to seek my help. He had no need to feel ashamed. If you fell overboard in the middle of the Atlantic, would you say to the person that was about to throw you a lifebelt: "Please don't, I don't want any help, I need to do this myself!"

If one of our teeth needed extracting, we wouldn't regard it as lack of will-power if we sought the assistance of an expert dentist and would regard it as crass stupidity to attempt to do it ourselves. Let's dispel the next misconception:

IT TAKES WILL-POWER TO QUIT

23

IT TAKES WILL-POWER TO QUIT

When I first discovered Easyway I naturally thought that my main adversary in the war against nicotine addiction would be the tobacco industry. Amazingly, even with its dubious motives and immense finances, the tobacco industry was preceded by several institutions that I believed would be my main allies. One is the body whose only purpose is to protect the public from misleading TV adverts. I have often been blamed because I've never advertised Easyway on national TV. I did try. This is a synopsis of the conversation I had with the authority concerned:

A: "We cannot accept this advert because you claim that your method doesn't require will-power to quit."
Me: "But it doesn't."
A: "Oh, come on, everyone knows it takes will-power to quit."
Me: "Are you an expert on helping smokers to quit?"
A: "No, not personally, but the rule was decided by an expert physician."
Me: "He's obviously not aware of Easyway. Would you please arrange an appointment with him so that I can explain why Easyway doesn't require the use of will-power."
A: "I'm sorry I can't do that, it's against the rules."
Me: "Would you give me his name?"
A: "Sorry, also against the rules. Anyway, everyone knows that it takes will-power to quit."
Me: "So you are an expert? Tell me, if you are walking along the road and have no desire to cross the road, does it take will-power not to cross the road?"
A: "What has this to do with quitting smoking?"
Me: " Easyway removes the desire to smoke before the smoker extinguishes his final cigarette. If he has no desire to smoke, why should it take will-power not to?"
A: "Look, we are wasting each other's time. There is no way you can break the rule, but I'm here to help you. All you need do is to amend your statement: you don't need will-power to: with the help of your will-power etc."
Me: "But your function is to protect the public from deception. Are you really advising me to tell lies? If the smoker has to use will-power, why would he need Easyway?"

They say fact is stranger than fiction. Can you believe that at a time when governments were insisting that health warnings appeared on cigarette packets, when they were overtly encouraging smokers to quit, they would allow the tobacco industry to spend tens of millions annually promoting their filth, yet ban Allen Carr from spending a comparative pittance advertising a method that would actually help smokers to escape, and then claim that body was acting in the public's interest?

Most smokers believe that they are weak-willed. Why is this? Because all smokers instinctively know that smoking is stupid and secretly want to quit. Why have they failed to quit? Because society has brainwashed us to believe that it takes will-power to quit.

This was one of the mysteries that I could never understand. I knew that I was a very strong-willed person. I wouldn't allow anyone to dominate me. I was in complete control of every other aspect of my life. I hated and despised myself for being completely dominated by nicotine.

Get it clearly into your mind that quitting has absolutely nothing to do with will-power. Will-power is something that you exercise against other things and other people. With smoking, it's not lack of will-power that keeps you smoking, but a conflict of wills. No one forces you to smoke but yourself. At our clinics we say to smokers who believe they are weak-willed: "If you ran out late at night, how far would you walk for a packet of cigarettes? A mile? Two miles?"

A smoker would swim the English Channel for a packet of cigarettes! On National No Smoking Days the media say: "This is the day that every smoker decides to quit."

In truth it is the one day in the year that smokers not only smoke twice as many as usual, but twice as blatantly as usual, because smokers resent being told what they can and can't do, particularly by the do-gooders who haven't the slightest notion of what smoking is about.

When the connection between smoking and lung cancer was first established, many smokers quit. That was because their fear of contracting lung cancer outweighed their fear of quitting. It takes a strong-willed person to block their minds to the health hazards, the waste of money, the slavery and the filth and stigma of being a smoker. It takes a particularly strong-willed person to resist the anti-social pressures that smokers are subjected to nowadays.

The man on the yacht was a classic example. He was neither a weak person nor weak-willed. Don't just take my word for it. Examine your own friends and relatives. You'll find that most heavy smokers are not only physically strong – you have to be physically strong to cope with the poison – but are dominant types. This is because the main illusion about smoking is that it relieves stress, and it is physically and mentally strong people that take on responsibility and stress.

It is this knowledge that we are both physically and mentally strong in other ways that leads us to believe another of the illusions:

I HAVE AN ADDICTIVE PERSONALITY

24

I HAVE AN ADDICTIVE PERSONALITY

We tend to divide the world into two distinct categories: them and us. Depending on our particular upbringing or prejudices, them and us can mean many different things, including male and female, black and white, rich and poor, Catholic and Protestant. I've always thought of myself as a fairminded person, and, with one notable exception, completely free of such prejudices. For me, there was only one significant distinction:

SMOKERS AND NON-SMOKERS

Non-smokers were an entirely different breed: boring, insipid, wishy-washy killjoys, the sort that if their toilet disinfectant would only kill 99 percent of all known germs, would spend the whole of their lives worrying about the other one percent, whereas smokers were exciting, interesting, dynamic, debonair, sociable types. Earlier I described the incident of the girl at a party, who had spent the whole night conversing with a man who could have been Dracula, all because he was the only smoker there. That was certainly my attitude.

If you analyze your smoking friends and colleagues, you will find that they do not appear stupid in other respects. As I have already explained, the main illusion about smoking is that it relieves stress and it is physically and mentally dominant types who tend to take on responsibility and stress. You'll find that heavy smokers tend to fall into this category, and casual smokers tend to have less stress in their lives. The man on the yacht was a classic example.

There is a smoking type and it is the same type that skis down mogul black runs and takes up hobbies like hang-gliding, bungy-jumping and motor racing. But there is no such thing as an addictive personality. It's the drug itself that addicts you. Most of my life I was convinced that I had an addictive personality. After all, I couldn't think of any rational reason why I couldn't quit. I knew it wasn't through lack of will-power, so there was only one logical explanation:

I HAD AN ADDICTIVE PERSONALITY

Many smokers of my generation experimented with joints. I've never taken a single puff of marijuana, let alone any harder drugs. So hooked was I on nicotine, so convinced that I had an addictive personality, I thought I'd be dead within a month if I dabbled with harder drugs.

What happened to my addictive personality once I discovered the mysteries of the nicotine trap? No one chooses to become a drug addict. We don't get hooked because we have addictive personalities. That would be like saying that people who got their foot caught in a bear trap had bear trap personalities. The type of person who spends his life walking through country that contains bear traps is obviously more likely to fall into the trap than one who spends his life in the metropolis.

Do you not think that it is an incredible coincidence that the only people who believe they have addictive personalities are people who become addicted to drugs?

IT'S THE DRUG THAT ADDICTS YOU – NOT YOUR PERSONALITY

Addictive drugs make you believe that you have an addictive personality. The distinction is important. You will never be completely free if you believe you have an addictive personality.

Now that I am free and can see the world as it is rather than through the drugged-up and panic-stricken brain of the addict, I find it difficult to believe that my view of non-smokers was so distorted. Most of my lifelong friends are non-smokers, my brother is a non-smoker, my wife is a non-smoker, the most dynamic and interesting people you could wish to meet.

In hindsight, I can only believe that I had this distorted view of non-smokers because smokers feel unclean and stupid in the presence of non-smokers. It's self protection. We sense that non-smokers despise us and search for excuses to avoid their company. This is why all drug addicts tend to huddle together.

Let's now tackle the next illusion. This is another matter that tends to make us believe that there is such a thing as an addictive personality:

DOES SMOKING HELP TO REDUCE WEIGHT?

25

DOES SMOKING HELP TO REDUCE WEIGHT?

Again, it does the complete opposite. Allow me to use my own experience as an example. When we wake up each morning, we immediately relieve certain aggravations, like our bladder and our thirst. Non-smokers will also relieve their hunger by eating breakfast.

Smokers will have an additional aggravation: they will have gone eight hours without nicotine. This is why the first cigarette of the day is a special one for many smokers. Ironically, it's also the one that tastes the worst, the one that makes us cough and splutter. It also helps to confirm that there is no genuine pleasure in smoking. The only illusion of pleasure is to partially relieve that empty, insecure feeling and since each cigarette, far from relieving it, simply continues the chain, there is no real pleasure.

That empty, insecure feeling is identical to a hunger for food. In the bad old days, before cancer scares, we neither had to discipline ourselves to eat breakfast before we lit up, nor was it regarded as anti-social to smoke in the bedroom. On the contrary. When I was in the army, it was common practice for everyone in the billet to smoke half a cigarette in bed after lights out, while we discussed obvious solutions to religious, political and sexual problems. In the mornings we would awake to the dawn chorus. No, I'm not referring to the birds; they were doing their best, but their harmonies were drowned out by the cacophony of coughing and spluttering when we lit the other half of that cigarette. I've said everyone. If I'm honest, there was usually one – possibly two – weirdos who inexplicably denied themselves the obvious 'pleasure' of that first cigarette.

Although the feeling of the little monster is identical to hunger for food, nicotine will not relieve a craving for food, or vice-versa. Because I hadn't eaten breakfast, I still had the empty feeling. This meant only one thing to my drugged brain: you need another cigarette. Any self-respecting smoker knows that if you are short of money and it's a choice between food and fags, there's only one winner.

Of course the second cigarette didn't relieve my hunger for food either, and like many smokers, I got out of the habit of eating breakfast. Eventually I stopped eating lunch as well. In fact, I would chain-smoke all day. I actually used to look forward to the end of a day's work just so that I could stop smoking for a while and give my lungs a rest.

Joyce would cook a large evening meal but I was still hungry. I was also addicted to oranges. I would eat orange after orange. The juice would be coming out of my mouth but I still wanted more. In fact, she used to say: "If ever I wanted to get rid of you, I'd just buy a sack of oranges and watch you explode." What I didn't realize then was that I had reversed the process. Now my body was craving nicotine and no matter how much food I stuffed into my mouth, the empty feeling would still be there.

I was a chain-smoker that didn't eat breakfast or lunch yet was still 28 pounds overweight. Smoking doesn't help to reduce weight; on the contrary, it creates an empty feeling. As your body becomes immune to the drug, you only partially relieve the feeling. This is what makes smokers turn to other drugs like alcohol, marijuana through to heroin, which reinforces this belief that certain people have addictive personalities.

If you take the trouble to research the matter, you will find that the vast majority of alcoholics are or were smokers and that the same applies to other drug addiction. When so-called experts say, "Oh, it's alright in moderation", they might just as well be saying, "Yes, by all means go over Niagara Falls, but don't go down more than a few feet."

Like the frog popped into boiling water, Niagara is obvious. But drugs are more subtle and cunning. Frogs like water, they particularly like warm water. Simmer a frog slowly and by the time it realizes that it wants to jump out, it also realizes that it can't. Drugs have the same softly, softly effect, with one difference – once you understand the confidence trick:

IT'S EASY TO QUIT

It is a fact that over 99 percent of alcoholics and heroin addicts are or were smokers. This might support the theory of addictive personalities. However, the majority of smokers do not become alcoholics or heroin addicts.

The main reason that we believe that smoking helps to reduce weight is that smokers who quit when using the 'will-power' method, tend to use substitutes like sweets or chocolates. Let me now explain why:

ALL SUBSTITUTES MAKE IT HARDER TO QUIT

26

ALL SUBSTITUTES MAKE IT HARDER TO QUIT

The most common and at the same time the most damaging substitutes involve NRT: gums, patches, nasal sprays containing nicotine. Why? Because they are legal, are promoted by massive TV advertising and have the support of the established medical profession. In theory, NRT sounds logical. When you try to quit smoking you have powerful enemies to defeat:

• To break the habit.
• To survive the terrible withdrawal symptoms.

Now, it doesn't take a top general to deduce that if you have two powerful enemies to defeat, only an idiot would attempt to take them on at the same time. So the theory is that you first stop smoking in order to break the habit but keep taking nicotine in another form in order to prevent the terrible withdrawal symptoms. Once you have successfully broken the habit, you then gradually wean yourself off the nicotine substitute.

Now, I cannot argue with the theory. It seems completely logical, but before I explain why it isn't, I would ask you to consider the following:

• Wouldn't it be even easier in theory to adopt the policy of the lady who cut out one cigarette each day. This way you would not only gradually wean yourself off the nicotine but you could also gradually break the habit. The fact is that most smokers discover sooner or later that, for the reasons I have already explained, cutting down, far from helping you off smoking, makes each cigarette appear to be more precious.
• NRT has been common knowledge for over 30 years. The same principles apply to patches and nasal sprays as the gum. If they worked, why would anyone still be smoking ?

I have asked countless qualified doctors who advocate NRT how you cure an addict of a drug by prescribing the same drug administered in another form. Not only have I never received one logical answer to that question, but not one qualified physician has ever even attempted to answer it. In fact, when I put the question, the reaction appears to be that they haven't even considered it, let alone thought of an answer to it.

NRT sounds logical, but it is based on the wrong facts:

• SMOKING ISN'T HABIT – IT'S DRUG ADDICTION!
• THE ACTUAL PHYSICAL WITHDRAWAL SYMPTOMS FROM NICOTINE ARE SO SLIGHT YOU DON'T NEED A SUBSTITUTE!

What are we trying to achieve? To stop smoking? No! To remove the desire to smoke. Nicotine replacement simply prolongs the life of the little monster. Even worse, while you prolong that empty feeling, you prolong the life of the big monster in your brain, whose only ambition is to satisfy the little monster!

All substitutes make it more difficult to quit, particularly NRT because it actually prolongs the life of both monsters. Other substitutes do the same. We might reason that we can't have a cigarette, so we'll substitute some other reward like a chocolate or chewing gum or whatever.

By simply going through that mental exercise you are telling yourself that you are making a sacrifice. Get it into your mind: before you fell into the nicotine trap you didn't need to smoke either to enjoy social occasions or to cope with stress. Smoking is an awful disease. I don't mean it causes awful diseases like lung cancer. I mean that simply being a nicotine addict is the worst disease you are ever likely to suffer from, unless you remain hooked, when you will suffer one or more of those other awful diseases.

When you get rid of a bout of flu, do you start searching for another disease to take its place? Of course you don't! You are just delighted to be rid of the disease. For a few days after the final cigarette the little monster will remind you: "You need a cigarette." If you say to yourself: "I can't have a cigarette so I'll have a toffee instead," you will simply prolong the process. The toffee won't placate the feeling anyway, so you will need another and another. Soon you will be utterly sick of toffees, you will have ruined your appetite for your main meals and you will be grossly overweight. You will have perpetuated the belief that what you really need is not the substitute but the real McCoy and eventually you will find an excuse to have a cigarette. I will explain later how to handle those times during which the little monster continues to trigger the need for a cigarette, so that they become moments of pleasure rather than misery.

Also remember that smokers who put on weight because they use substitutes do so not because they stopped smoking but because they started. The same applies to any other slight aggravation you might experience when quitting. Non-smokers do not suffer from these problems.

We've now reached the stage where we have removed all the illusions but two:

19. Is it necessary to suffer from withdrawal symptoms when quitting?
20. Is it difficult to quit?

However, both matters are best dealt with during the instructions prior to the ritual of the final cigarette. There are two important matters which take precedence. First:

THE INCREDIBLE PLEASURE OF BEING A NON-SMOKER!

27

THE INCREDIBLE PLEASURE OF BEING
A NON-SMOKER

You have probably noticed that whenever society discusses the question of smokers permanently abstaining, they invariably refer to: 'giving up'. You might also have noticed that I always refer to stopping or quitting and never refer to 'giving up'. The reason is that the mere expression implies that we are making a sacrifice:

THERE IS NO SACRIFICE! THERE IS NOTHING TO GIVE UP!

This is difficult for smokers to believe; nevertheless it is true. At our clinics the most common reason that smokers give for quitting is health. Money comes a very poor second and is almost an afterthought. Health was certainly the reason I desperately wanted to quit. Money never even entered into the equation; surprising when you consider the thousands I spent on tobacco.

The 'Moment of Revelation' was by far the most exhilarating moment of my life and at that time it seemed inconceivable that I would receive four other gains which to me were more precious than health or money. Any billionaire suffering from a terminal disease knows that health is the most important thing in life and would sacrifice all his billions for good health. No one would argue with that fact. Equally you cannot argue with the fact that smokers do knowingly risk awful diseases.

I knew that my permanent cough and my regular attacks of asthma and bronchitis were directly due to smoking, but like the simmering frog, I was used to it, I could handle it and I knew no better. But what I didn't realize was that my permanent state of lethargy was also caused by smoking.

As a teenager I was a physical fitness fanatic. I can remember rushing around for the sheer joy of it. But from my early 20s I struggled to get up at 9am. For years I felt permanently tired. In the evenings I would lie on a sofa watching TV half asleep. Because my father was the same, I thought that was normal. I truly believed that old age started in the late 20s.

A few days after quitting, I started to wake up at 7am feeling completely rested and energetic. I actually wanted to exercise, jog, swim and play tennis. The extra energy is a wonderful bonus. I'd forgotten the sheer joy of bursting with energy.

However, there were three other bonuses that I wasn't expecting to receive. The sheer slavery of being a smoker had never dawned on me. Like the man on the yacht, I'd spent so much of my life defending my right to kill myself, resisting all the pressures from society trying to force me to quit, it never dawned on me that non-smokers don't have this problem of worrying whether this office, this flight or this building is smoking or non-smoking.

In the bad old days you could visit a friend or stranger's house – it didn't bother you whether they were smokers or non-smokers. You'd say: "Do you mind if I smoke?" It was really a polite way of asking for an ashtray. Nowadays you hope to see an ashtray, and if you pluck up the courage to ask: "Do you mind if I smoke?", the occupant will look at you with the same expression as if you had said: "I'm hungry, do you mind if I eat your goldfish?" Ask for an ashtray and they'll reply: "An ashtray? No, I'm awfully sorry. Do you mind smoking in the garden?"

Please bear in mind that this slavery will get worse and worse. Every week smokers are being attacked by some faction of society. Like the man on the yacht, stop resisting it.

For me, the second biggest gain that came from quitting was to be free of the self-despising. All our lives as smokers we know instinctively that we have fallen into an evil trap. We try to block our minds to it, but it is like an ever increasing dark cloud at the back of our minds. Smokers, particularly heavy smokers, do tend to be physically and mentally dominant types. Dominant people hate to be ruled by anyone or anything. I cannot begin to describe just how lovely it is to be free, to realize that there is no weakness in you, to be able to look at smokers, not with a feeling of envy because you are no longer allowed to smoke, but with a feeling of genuine pity as you would look at a heroin addict.

Perhaps I'm giving the impression that I feel superior and look down on smokers. Not so. What I'm actually saying is how nice it is no longer to feel inferior or to despise yourself and how nice it is to have self-respect.

However, the greatest gain I received from quitting was the return of my confidence and courage. It was blatantly obvious that smoking was killing me physically, but I was convinced it gave me confidence and courage. There used to be a brand of cigarettes named 'Strand'. The advertising slogan was:

YOU ARE NEVER ALONE WITH A STRAND

I never smoked Strand but that was my attitude to cigarettes. They were my confidence, my courage, my very character and personality. Provided I had a packet of cigarettes in my pocket, I didn't need anything or anyone else. If you believe that, which I once did, it's not surprising that we feel so miserable, deprived and insecure when we try to quit.

As a teenager, I was proud of my body. The thought that something could go wrong with it never even occurred to me. I thought I was indestructible. I used to enjoy medical examinations at school. My attitude to the doctor was: see if you can find something wrong. In my 20s I began to hate medicals. I refused to have life insurance. I would say to my wife: "We can't afford it". It wasn't that, it was because I couldn't bear the thought of a medical. In fact, the thought of chest X-rays filled me with horror.

Just as I blamed my lack of energy on old age, so I blamed my loss of courage and confidence on old age. It never dawned on me that nicotine addiction was not only destroying me physically, but was also destroying my courage and confidence.

When you feel both physically and mentally low, you seem to have all the problems in the world. The slightest set-back is the straw that breaks the camel's back. I'd reached the stage where I was so low physically and mentally that I thought: "If this is life with my little crutch, I cannot bear the thought of life without it." However, when you feel energetic and strong both physically and mentally, problems cease to be problems; they simply become part of the exciting challenge of life. Life is wonderful. It is meant to be exciting.

I could understand why smokers blocked their minds to diseases like lung cancer, heart disease, strokes, emphysema and thrombosis. We think it's like playing Russian Roulette: you were either unlucky or you got away with it.

However, I could never understand arteriosclerosis. I'd heard about these cranks that were warned that if they didn't quit, their circulation would become so bad that gangrene would set in in their fingers and toes. Could you believe that any smoker would be stupid enough to continue smoking faced with that ultimatum?

Well, perhaps they thought the doctor was bluffing. But then having had their toes removed and being threatened with the loss of their feet and eventually their legs:

THEY STILL DIDN'T QUIT!

Do you write off these smokers as a few fanatical cranks as I used to? If so, open your mind, you are suffering from exactly the same disease! These people aren't cranks. The explanation that makes them lose their legs rather than quit smoking is fear – that panic feeling created by the little monster. That's what makes us block our minds to the evils of smoking.

That feeling is real and the lower it drags you down physically and mentally, the greater your need for the illusion of the slight boost when you light up. That feeling is caused by the cigarette, and the greatest gain you'll receive from quitting is to be free of that empty, insecure feeling and the loss of confidence and courage that goes with it.

The greatest evil about smoking is that by destroying you physically and mentally you lose:

THE JOY OF LIVING!

That's why I want you to quit, not because it's killing you and costing you a fortune, but because I want you to share with me the incredible joy of living. Fifteen years ago I was a cynical old man ready to die. Today at the age of 64 I feel like a young boy looking forward to each day. I probably won't live to be 100. It doesn't bother me one way or the other. I'm just so happy to be alive now and enjoying life. I want you to quit for the purely selfish reason that:

LIFE IS SO MUCH MORE ENJOYABLE AS A NON-SMOKER!

I have stated that Easyway does not involve shock treatment. This is because if you tell a smoker that smoking kills them, it creates panic. What is the first thing that smokers do when they feel anxious? They light a cigarette. If you haven't yet decided that you are going to quit, then skip the next chapter and come back to it when you have made the decision to quit. If you have already made the decision to quit, the next chapter will not be shock treatment to you, but will confirm that you have made the correct decision:

HEALTH

28

HEALTH

I am not trying to underplay the effects of the killer diseases. Our loved ones cannot understand why we torture them by risking our health and their peace of mind. It is because we are like the simmering frog. We never consciously made the decision to get hooked. We know we will stop one day, but not today. In the meantime what's the point of torturing ourselves by thinking about such horrors? We get into the habit of blocking our minds to them.

You've now decided that you want to quit. So let's start using these facts to help you quit easily and permanently. Did you see the film *The Deer Hunter*? Can you remember the horror of the scene in which two of the characters play Russian Roulette? Would you be stupid enough to play Russian Roulette? Doctors now state that one in two smokers die as a direct result of their smoking. It's widely accepted that the odds are at least one in three. That's worse odds than Russian Roulette.

But Russian Roulette kills you immediately, smoking takes years. Does that really make a difference? If you knew that the next cigarette would trigger off cancer in your lungs, do you think you would smoke that cigarette? Smoking is a chain reaction. When you lit that first cigarette, you lit a fuse that is slowly burning away and will one day explode inside your body. There is no way of knowing the length of that fuse. If you continue to keep your head in the sand, you will be as stupid as the man who, having fallen from the roof of a skyscraper and hurtling past the tenth floor, says to himself: "So far so good".

If you feel stupid being a smoker now, just think how many times more stupid you will feel if you do leave it too late. My profession regularly brings me into contact with people who leave it too late. Awful as those diseases are, the worst thing that happens to those smokers is not the disease itself, but the knowledge that they left it too late. When that happens to them, the lifetime's brainwashing about the glamour and pleasures of smoking are reversed instantaneously.

PLEASE DON'T LET THAT HAPPEN TO YOU!
HOW WILL YOU FACE YOUR LOVED ONES IF YOU DO?

Stop saying: "It won't happen to me." Thereby ensuring that it does! Use this information to help keep you a happy non-smoker. Start thinking: "It will happen to me."

THEREBY ENSURING THAT IT DOESN'T!

I'm convinced that if I could have seen what was happening inside my body, I would not have continued to smoke. I am now referring to this regular and progressive gunging up of our circulatory system. It wouldn't be quite so bad if we just starved every cell in our body of oxygen and other nutrients, but we actually replace that shortage with numerous poisonous compounds such as nicotine, carbon monoxide, tars and many others.

It's bad enough that this starvation process causes shortage of breath and a feeling of lethargy, but its most serious effect is that it prevents every organ and muscle of our bodies from operating efficiently. It has a similar effect to AIDS. It gradually destroys our immune system. Many doctors are now relating all sorts of diseases to smoking, including diabetes, cervical cancer and breast cancer. Several of the adverse effects that smoking had on my health, some of which I had been suffering from for years, did not become apparent to me until many years after I had quit.

It didn't even occur to me that for years I was on the way to arteriosclerosis. My almost permanently grey complexion I explained as natural to me or attributed to lack of exercise. It never occurred to me that it was really due to the blocking up of my capillaries. I had varicose veins in my thirties which have miraculously disappeared since I stopped smoking. I reached the stage about five years before I stopped when every night I would have this weird sensation in my legs. I would get Joyce to massage my legs every night. It didn't occur to me until at least a year after I had stopped that I no longer needed the massage. About two years before I quit, I would occasionally get violent pains in my chest, which I feared must be lung cancer but now assume to have been angina. I haven't had any attacks since I quit.

When I was a child I would bleed profusely from cuts. This frightened me. I suspected that I was a haemophiliac and feared that I might bleed to death. Later in life I would sustain quite deep cuts yet hardly bleed at all. A browny-red gunge would ooze from the cut.

This worried me. I knew that blood was meant to be bright red and I assumed that I had some sort of blood disease. However, I was pleased about the consistency which meant that I no longer bled profusely. Not until after I had stopped smoking did I learn that smoking thickens the blood and that the brownish hue was due to lack of oxygen. I was ignorant of the effect at the time but, in hindsight, it was this effect that smoking was having on my health that most fills me with horror. When I think of my poor heart trying to pump that gunge around restricted blood vessels – day in, day out – without missing a single beat, I find it a miracle that I didn't suffer a stroke or a heart attack. It made me realize not how fragile our bodies are but how strong and ingenious that incredible machine is! I've always ensured that the oil and filters in my car are regularly changed. I still find it incredible that I was so meticulous about my car and at the same time completely oblivious to the daily damage that I deliberately inflicted on the vehicle on which my very survival depended.

I had liver spots on my hands in my forties. I tried to ignore them, assuming that they were due to early senility caused by the hectic lifestyle that I had led. It was two years after I had quit that a smoker at one of our clinics remarked that when he had stopped previously, his liver spots disappeared. I had forgotten about mine; to my amazement, they too had disappeared.

As long as I can remember, I had spots flashing in front of my eyes if ever I stood up too quickly, particularly out of the bathtub. I would feel dizzy as if I were about to black out. I never related this to smoking. In fact, I was convinced that it was quite normal and that everyone else had similar effects. Not until three years after I had quit, when an ex-smoker told me that he no longer had that sensation, did it occur to me that I no longer had it either.

You might conclude that I am somewhat of a hypochondriac. I believe that I was when I was a smoker. One of the great evils about smoking is that it fools us into believing that nicotine gives us courage, when in fact it gradually and imperceptibly dissipates it. I was shocked when I heard my father say that he had no wish to live to be fifty. Little did I realize that 20 years later I would have exactly the same lack of joy of living. You might conclude that this chapter has been one of necessary, or unnecessary, doom and gloom. I promise you it is the complete opposite. I used to fear death when I was a child. I used to believe that smoking removed that fear. Perhaps it did. If so, it replaced it with something infinitely worse:

A FEAR OF LIVING!

Now my fear of dying has returned. It does not bother me. I realize that it only exists because I now enjoy life so much. I don't brood over my fear of dying any more than I did when I was a child. I'm far too busy living my life to the full. The odds are against my living to a hundred, but I'll try to. I'll also try to enjoy every precious moment!

There were two other advantages on the health side that never occurred to me until I had stopped smoking. One was that I used to have nightmares every night. I can only assume that these nightmares were the result of the body being deprived of nicotine throughout the night and the insecure feeling that would result. Now the only nightmare is that I occasionally dream that I am smoking again. This is quite a common dream among ex-smokers. Some worry that it means that they are still subconsciously pining for a cigarette. Don't worry about it. The fact that it was a nightmare means that you are very pleased not to be a smoker. There is that twilight zone with any nightmare when you wake up and are not sure whether it is a genuine catastrophe. Isn't it wonderful when you realize that it was only a dream? We are nearly there now. There is just one more important subject matter to discuss before you smoke that final cigarette:

THE VOID

29

THE VOID

There were two powerful pieces of evidence that helped me to see clearly through the mysteries and miseries of smoking. One was reflecting back on my life before I became hooked, the drabness of my life for the years that I was hooked and how the joy of living has returned since I quit. It was like going from Technicolor to black and white and back to Technicolor. The black and white period started when I got hooked and ended the moment I knew I was free. Throughout all three periods I enjoyed the genuine highs and coped with the genuine lows that life provides. In all the thousands of 'thank you' letters that I have received, perhaps the most common statement is:

THANK YOU FOR GIVING ME BACK MY LIFE!

People don't mean thank you for preventing my contracting some awful disease, but thank you for helping me out of the nightmare into the sunshine! The strength of the human body combined with the power of the human brain makes us the most sophisticated and powerful survival machine on the planet. I'm not just referring to myself but to every human fortunate enough to be born with a body and brain that isn't defective. Whether you believe that we were created by a god, or are the result of 3 billion years of evolution and natural selection, or a combination of both, cannot alter the fact that, on planet Earth, human beings are the pinnacle of creation. The fact that my heart was able to pump that gunge through restricted blood vessels for a third of a century without missing a single beat, proves how incredibly strong the human body is.

Youngsters nowadays all seem to be searching for some magic pill as if the Creator and the 3 billion years of trial and error have produced a dud, or that some important ingredient is missing.

We believe that we lead stressful lives. It's nonsense. In Western society we have eliminated genuine stress. When we leave our homes we don't live in fear of being attacked by wild animals and most of us don't have to worry where our next meal will come from or whether we'll have a roof for the night. Powerful businessmen ask me: "How will I be able to answer a phone without a cigarette?" What is so stressful about a phone? It won't blow up or bite them. Their stress is caused by nicotine.

Think of the life of wild animals. A rabbit isn't even safe in its burrow. Its entire life is survival and it survives! It has adrenalin and other drugs. So do we! The human body is an incredibly complicated survival machine a million times more sophisticated and complicated than the most intelligent and educated human beings can possibly comprehend. Our brains automatically supply our bodies with the drugs we need as and when we need them. That's how wild animals have survived for millions of years without the benefit of drugs, stores of food, clothes, fire or doctors, and that's how the human race survived on the planet for over 99.99 percent of its existence. To interfere with that incredibly sophisticated machine by introducing drugs and poisons is about as sensible as thinking your pet gorilla could repair your TV.

At the other end of the scale smokers ask: "How can I possibly enjoy life without a cigarette?" Watch children at a birthday party. The boys arrive in their Sunday clothing, shy and inhibited; butter wouldn't melt in their mouths. Five minutes later they are destroying the place. They are on a complete high. They don't need nicotine, alcohol or any other poison:

A TRUE HIGH IS JUST FEELING GREAT TO BE ALIVE!

Not only are we brainwashed from birth to believe that smoking provides some sort of pleasure or crutch, but we are also brainwashed to believe that we are incomplete, that we need some outside prop or drug.

School-days are purported to be the best days of our lives. It's only adults who seem to think so. In fact, for all creatures on this planet it's the complete reverse. The most stressful period in our lives is birth, gradually decreasing through childhood and adolescence. Stress should end with maturity. We are brainwashed to believe that stress should increase as we get older.

The problem is that during the genuinely stressful period of adolescence, we get hooked on illusory crutches and, as they drag us down physically and mentally, our problems appear to get increasingly worse. The result is that we never feel completely mature or secure. I didn't feel complete security until I escaped from the nicotine trap. I can appreciate that old age combined with ill health could be genuinely stressful. All I can tell you is that I felt old in my 30s. In my mid-60s I feel like a young boy. I'm fortunate to be blessed with good health. I hope it lasts. Either way, I'm not going to worry about it.

It is not only essential to remove the brainwashing that smoking provides some form or pleasure or crutch, it is even more important to remove the belief that we are incomplete, that there is a void in our lives. Youngsters aren't getting hooked nowadays because they are stupid, but because they are brainwashed to believe that they are incomplete. Is it surprising that they experiment with what we have also brainwashed them to believe are the least harmful chemicals: nicotine and alcohol? After all, so many adults are still using them and claiming that they are in control.

Let me now use a couple of examples. A few years ago I was at a dinner party. There was a girl there I had met once before, but she had got embarrassed smoking in my presence; people know what I do for my living and assume that I'll lecture them. It so happened that on this second occasion, she was the only smoker there, but even though the meal had finished, she wasn't smoking but had 'the smoker's twitch'. She sat fiddling with her lighter. I cannot bear to see smokers in that position and said: "Margaret, the meal is over, no one will complain, have a cigarette if you need one." She said: "I don't need one, but I would like one." I should have shut up really, but it was like waving a red rag under my nose. I said: "If you don't need one, leave it. There's no point in choking yourself if you don't need to." She was about to light up. Instead she just said: "Fine, I'll leave it." I was talking to another girl who I hadn't met before, but my attention remained with Margaret. I wanted to see how she would get over the situation and of course now the twitching became unbearable.

I was now beginning to feel petty. Far from easing the situation, I had made it worse. I was trying to think of a way to get over the impasse, when the girl that I had been chatting to suddenly said: "I'd murder for a cigarette now." I was truly shaken, because I was convinced the girl was a non-smoker. I said: "I'm sorry, I didn't realize you were a smoker. Please don't worry about me, I was the the world's worst." She said: "No way! I haven't smoked for eight years, and I will never smoke again. But I used to love a cigarette after a meal and I really would enjoy one now." Meanwhile Margaret, who believed I was now genuinely occupied with the vicar's wife, had lit up and was taking a sneaky drag.

The incident amply illustrates the total futility of being a smoker. There was Margaret, looking decidedly guilty and uncomfortable, snatching sneaky puffs on her cigarette, hoping that no one had noticed that she had lit up and wishing she were free like everyone else in the room. The other girl was being even more ridiculous. She had obviously quit because, for whatever reason, she didn't like being a smoker. What's the point of saying: "I want to be a non-smoker," and then spending the rest of your life at odd times craving for something that:

YOU SINCERELY HOPE YOU WILL NEVER HAVE!

so that you spend the rest of your life feeling deprived and miserable? Because the majority of smokers who quit by using some variation of the 'will-power' method do this, we assume that it's natural to go on doing it. No, they only do it because they genuinely believe that cigarettes did improve a meal.

However, the thing that I would really like you to get into your mind is not only are they moping for something that they hope they will never have, but they never,

ever had it in the first place. Complaining ex-smokers will say to non-smokers: "It's alright for you, you've never been a smoker, so you don't know what you're missing." It doesn't seem to occur to the smoker that there wasn't ever anything to miss!

It's important to remove this part of the brainwashing, about those so-called 'special' cigarettes after a meal. You've had thousands and thousands of meals in your life, but how many of those precious cigarettes do you remember smoking? Think back on your life: when you allowed yourself to smoke as and when you wanted to, didn't you take those cigarettes for granted? Aren't all the memories you retain about the early days when they made you feel sick? Or like the man on the yacht, when you had run out of cigarettes or were running low? Or when you were trying to cut down and they dominated your whole life? Or when you were trying to quit and felt miserable and deprived?

Easyway is designed to make it easy and enjoyable to quit. It is also designed to keep you a happy non-smoker permanently. You might have already discerned that I do what I do not through altruistic motives, but because I get tremendous pleasure in helping fellow prisoners escape from the nicotine trap. Regrettably there is still one black cloud on my horizon. It is the smokers that send me lovely letters thanking me for helping them to escape, explaining how wonderful their lives are now that they have escaped and ending with the positive declaration that they will never, ever smoke another cigarette. What's so bad about that? The fact that some of them fall into the trap again.

The sceptical will say: "Obviously they weren't completely cured, otherwise why would they start again? It simply proves the theory: once a smoker always a smoker!" No, they were completely free, but smoking is an ingenious, subtle trap and you just need one mistake to fall back into it again. One of the problems of finding it easy to quit is that you lose the fear of being hooked again. You become like the youngster you were in the first place: "There's no harm in the odd cigarette, there's no way I could get hooked again, particularly now Allen Carr has explained the mystery of the trap." Allen Carr might explain why it would be stupid to put your neck on a chopping block, but if you are stupid enough to do so, don't blame me if you lose your head.

One of the reasons why smokers get hooked again is that although they fully understand that smoking does nothing for them whatsoever, they fail to remove the feeling of a void. There are four classic examples of occasions when smokers tend to get hooked again and, typically of the nicotine trap, they are the usual opposites: relaxation, stress, concentration and boredom. Let's use an example of each, starting with stress. I wonder how many thousands of smokers have started smoking again as the result of a road accident?

Let's assume that you are still a smoker, driving your wife to a restaurant to meet friends you haven't seen for several years. Suddenly the lights change and you brake rather sharply. No sooner have you done so than the car behind you drives into your brand new Porsche. OK, I was only fantasizing, so let's be realistic: it's a three-year-old Ford. Nevertheless, it's your pride and joy. You start shouting at the other driver. He starts shouting at you. It doesn't really matter who's right or wrong. Either way your pleasant evening has turned into a disaster.

Now, you must have had similar situations in your life. It doesn't really matter whether it was a road accident. But think back. Was your attitude: "Not only am I soaking wet and my evening has been ruined, but so has my beautiful car. I've now got to go through the trauma of insurance claims and repair shops, but who cares? I've got this glorious packet of cigarettes." Can you remember a single genuine tragedy in your life that was cured by the fact that you smoked a cigarette – other than the tragedy of being low or without cigarettes? If smoking relieved genuine tragedies, smokers would never suffer from genuine tragedies.

Now imagine that you've happily quit smoking for several months and the same thing happens. You are still going to feel miserable. It is very possible that someone will offer you a cigarette at such times. It might even occur to you that, at times like this, you would have had a cigarette, true:

BUT IT DIDN'T HELP

However, if you start moping for one now, only two things can happen: you either resist the temptation and feel even more miserable because you won't allow yourself to have one, or you make yourself even more miserable and fall back into the trap.

Accept that you are going to have tragedies in the future. If and when they come, instead of torturing yourself by moping for a situation that never ever existed, reinforce your joy of being a non-smoker. Remind yourself that whatever genuine tragedies happen to smokers, they are even lower because of the effects of being a smoker and remember how lucky you are to be free.

The second and most common example of smokers getting hooked again are social occasions. The worst thing that smokers do to non-smokers at social occasions is to put nicotine into the atmosphere. The reason that nicotine is the most addictive drug known to mankind is that you don't have to smoke it yourself to get hooked. Many non-smokers like the smell of certain tobaccos without ever having smoked themselves. In the bad old days when every living room and restaurant was saturated with cigarette smoke, even non-smokers were partially addicted.

It happens to our therapists after a group session involving heavy smokers. I can actually feel the empty, insecure feeling of the nicotine leaving my body. I know the little monster has been revived because occasionally I get the whiff of a cigarette or cigar and it smells gorgeous. This worries some people. They say: "Doesn't that make you want to smoke again?" I say: "On the contrary, I love the smell of a rose but I've no desire to smoke it. I'm just grateful that it's some other idiot that is having to breathe the filth into their lungs."

This is why ex-smokers are more aggressive to smokers than people who have never smoked. Non-smokers just pity smokers and tolerate them as you would a heroin addict. But when ex-smokers start breathing in the nicotine at social occasions, they are tempted to light up and to relieve the feeling. They know that if they do, they'll become hooked again. They also know that they are better off than the smokers. But the smokers don't seem to realize this, they seem happy and cheerful. It's self-protection: by attacking the smokers and telling them what a filthy, disgusting habit it is, ex-smokers are really reassuring themselves that they've made the right decision.

If you are worried that you might become one of these self-righteous ex-smokers, don't be; soon you will be genuinely pitying them as you would an alcoholic or a heroin addict. But always be aware that the brainwashing continues. When you have been free for several years, you might find yourself on vacation with a crowd of smokers. They are laughing and happy. The cigarettes are handed round. They are all doing something but you are no longer allowed to.

Just as the expression 'giving up' implies sacrifice, so the expression 'ex-smoker' can imply 'no longer allowed to smoke'. Remember those smokers aren't happy because they are smoking but because they are on vacation. Non-smokers enjoy vacations and social occasions. If you wanted to spoil their joy you could raise the subject and the majority of them would openly admit that they envy you. Some will feel too stupid to admit the fact and will try to justify their stupidity like you and I used to do. Anyway, there's no need to spoil their evening; just feel happy and safe in the knowledge that the biggest idiot on earth wouldn't choose to become a smoker and every one of those smokers will be envying you, whether they have the sense to admit it or not.

If you make the mistake of envying those smokers, you will simply make yourself miserable by moping for an illusion. Even worse, you might make yourself more miserable by starting the chain again. Instead use the moment to remind youself how nice it is to be free!

The third factor that tends to get us hooked again when we attempt to quit is the inability to concentrate. Smokers who quit by the 'will-power' method find it almost impossible to concentrate. This is because they genuinely believe that smoking helps them to concentrate, so the first time they have a mental block, their brains are programmed to think: "I really need a cigarette to help me concentrate." But they can't have one. Rather than concentrating on the mental block, their brains obsess about a completely different problem: the fact that for the rest of their lives they will be deprived of a genuine aid to concentration. And, of course, while their brains are obsessing, it's little wonder they are unable to overcome the mental block.

This was invariably the cause of my downfall whenever I attempted to quit by using the 'will-power' method. Amazingly, when I finally quit, I didn't suffer with lack of concentration in any way. This is because I knew that, far from aiding concentration, smoking actually impedes it. So now when I get mental blocks, I don't punish myself by moping for something that would actually impede my concentration. I do what non-smokers do when they have mental blocks and what I used to do before I fell into the nicotine trap: I try to overcome it, or have a break, or sleep on it or seek help.

I've explained how nicotine addiction creates the illusion that cigarettes help you to concentrate. If smoking genuinely did that, smokers would never get mental blocks or loss of memory. Can I claim that during the third of a century that I smoked that I never once suffered from a mental block or loss of memory? Obviously not. If smoking indeed provided these magical powers, university authorities would make it compulsory for all students to smoke. Interviewers for any job that involved concentration would insist that the applicants smoked. Such a notion is silly. If so, the very notion that smoking helps people to concentrate is equally nuts.

By far the most common example of ex-smokers falling into the trap again through boredom is caused by extended flight delays at airports. I'm not sure that it is just coincidence at such times, but you will always find yourself surrounded by attractive packs of duty-free cigarettes. The temptation is: "I'll just buy one pack just to get me over the delay." Don't! Instead think back to the time when you were a smoker and had similar delays. Were you happy and cheerful? If you need further proof, just look around at the smokers on the same flight and ask yourself whether they look happy and cheerful!

We've finally arrived at:

THE INSTRUCTIONS LEADING UP TO THE FINAL CIGARETTE

30

THE INSTRUCTIONS LEADING UP TO THE FINAL CIGARETTE

Does the thought of never having another cigarette fill you with panic? If so, try to face up to the only alternative:

NEVER EVER BEING ALLOWED TO QUIT

Perhaps you feel that the time is not quite right. Don't fall for it. Remember, one of the ingenuities of the trap is to make you keep putting it off. Also remember that you didn't decide to become a smoker. You spent all that precious money to choke yourself because you were conned. For years you were being controlled by something evil.

See smoking as it really is: a deadly, contagious, disease that progressively gets worse and worse. The time to get rid of that disease is now. Perhaps you've got a stressful period coming up or an exciting social occasion like a wedding. So much the better. You can prove to yourself immediately that you can cope with the stress and enjoy the social occasion without smoking.

There is no need to feel miserable or anxious. If you have butterflies in your stomach, remember that so do players when they come out for any world final – it's because you are about to achieve something wonderful. I've achieved several wonderful things in my life, including helping thousands of other smokers to quit. But the greatest achievement was my personal escape, and most of those other smokers tell me it was also theirs.

Perhaps you feel that the sense of achievement will be less because you didn't do it alone. I assure you it won't. Perhaps you can remember the thrill when you first swam without inflatables, or could ride your bicycle or passed your driving test. Was that sense of achievement less because you had help? We all need help.

If you feel the need, feel free to have a second-to-last cigarette while you are reading these instructions. When you light the final cigarette, do it not with an attitude of: "I musn't ever smoke another, or I'll never be allowed to smoke again", but of:

ISN'T IT WONDERFUL! I'M FREE! I'M A NON-SMOKER!

For a few days you will have a saboteur inside your body that will be starving and doing its best to undermine your resolution. I'm referring to the little nicotine monster. You might only recognize the feeling as an empty, insecure feeling. You might feel disoriented for a while. If so, just accept it, but don't worry about it, it will soon go.

Any change in life leaves us somewhat disoriented for a while, even improvements like a better job, house or car. For a few days the controls seem strange. We put the windshield wipers on when we mean to indicate. It's Sod's law: every time you change your car they switch them over. Also remember that any slight inconvenience you might experience is not because you quit smoking, but because you started:

NON-SMOKERS DON'T SUFFER FROM NICOTINE WITHDRAWAL!

Hey, wait a minute. Didn't I promise that with Easyway you won't suffer from withdrawal symptoms? Haven't I also implied that nicotine withdrawal is so bad that smokers would rather have their legs removed than quit? Get it clearly into your mind that the actual physical withdrawal from nicotine is so mild that we don't even realize it is there. That's what you suffer the whole of your smoking life. You will be no worse off when you extinguish the final cigarette. We only know that feeling as:

I WANT A CIGARETTE

What makes people have their legs removed and smokers suffer misery when they use the 'will-power' method to quit, is that they don't realize that the feeling is caused by the little monster. They believe that they want a cigarette because it is their crutch, their courage, their confidence and that they won't be able to cope with life or enjoy life without it.

"But you tell me that the little monster dies after about three weeks. Surely smokers using the 'will-power' method would feel free after three weeks of abstinence. Why aren't they?" Because that feeling is identical to normal hunger and normal stress. So even when the little monster has died, whenever the ex-smoker suffers normal hunger or stress, their brains still interpret the feeling as:

I WANT A CIGARETTE

Now you might have that feeling for a few days. If you do, be prepared for it, but don't worry about it. For convenience I sometimes describe the little monster as craving nicotine. The little monster is incapable of craving nicotine or anything else. It is only your brain that is capable of craving. Some so-called experts believe that it is essential to survive a transitional period of misery after you cut off the supply of nicotine before the ex-smoker ceases to crave nicotine. That is not so. Provided you follow all the instructions, you will be in complete control and will never, ever crave another cigarette.

Accept that you might have the feeling of: "I want a cigarette" for a few days after you have cut off the supply of nicotine. Don't worry about it and don't get into a panic. Just pause and say to yourself: "I know what this feeling is. I suffered it all my smoking life. It's not a pleasant feeling. It's a feeling of fear and insecurity. This is the feeling that makes smokers want a cigarette. It's caused by that little nicotine monster. It started with my first cigarette and was perpetuated by every subsequent cigarette. Isn't it wonderful? It's dying, I'm free!"

"But if it's identical to normal hunger and normal stress, how will I ever know when I'm free?" Because if you follow the instructions and understand the nature of the trap, you are already free the moment you cut off the supply of nicotine.

"Should I try not to think about smoking?" No! The biggest mistake that smokers make when using the 'will-power' method is to try not to think about smoking. If I say to you now: "Don't think of elephants!" What have you started to think about? And the only reason that you are thinking about them now is because I told you not to. It's like if you have a big day coming up. You think: I need a good night's sleep so I'll get to bed an hour earlier. If ever you've done that you'll know that the one thing you won't be able to do is sleep and the more you worry about it, the more you make certain it doesn't happen.

How can you not think about smoking? It's all around you and unless you help me to free the rest of the world quickly, it will be all around you for a few more years. In any event, the little monster will ensure that you think about it for the next few days. I think about it for 90 percent of my life. Why should you even not want to think about it? There's nothing bad happening. On the contrary, there's something wonderful happening. Don't worry if your whole mind is obsessed with it for the next few days. If you'd just won the lottery, wouldn't your mind be obsessed with the thought for a few days?

It's what you are thinking that is important. If you are thinking: "Oh, I'd love a cigarette but I'm not allowed to have one, or when will this craving end and I'll be free?", of course you will be miserable. But if you are thinking:

ISN'T IT GREAT I'M ALREADY FREE!

You'll feel great every time you think about smoking, and the more you think about it the better you will feel. "But how can I guarantee that I'll always think that way?"

By seeing smoking as it really is. If a close friend or relative dies you have to go through a period of mourning. You hope time will help heal the wound, but it never does completely. At odd times in the future you will remember and feel sad and nostalgic. This is what happens when smokers, alcoholics and other drug addicts 'give up'. They know they'll be better off if they can get free. But they do believe that they've lost a friend or crutch. However, the cigarette isn't dead and they remain vulnerable and can too easily get hooked again.

But if an enemy dies, you don't have to go through a period of mourning. You can rejoice immediately and you can go on rejoicing for the rest of your life. It's your choice. When you extinguish that final cigarette, you can spend the next few days moping that you no long suffer from the worst disease that you ever suffered from and be miserable. You might even abstain for a few days. Personally, I can't see any point in that, can you? Or you can spend the next few days and the rest of your life like me:

EXHILARATED THAT YOU ARE FREE FROM THE NICOTINE TRAP!

You don't need me to tell you that you have made the correct decision.

THERE ARE NO ADVANTAGES TO BEING A SMOKER WHATSOEVER! THERE ARE ONLY AWFUL DISADVANTAGES!

That's why nobody ever decided to become a smoker. Nicotine addiction, like all drug addiction, is a sinister, ingenious trap that is designed to keep you trapped for life unless you take positive steps to escape. You are in a wonderful position today. You fell into the trap, but you don't have to remain in it until it destroys you. What you are actually deciding today is not whether you are going to stop smoking, but whether you are going to spend the rest of your life as a smoker or a non-smoker.

Now, you and I are in no doubt that the people that love you will be ecstatic when you quit. If you still have doubts, I swear to you that the person who will be most ecstatic is you.

The second largest mistake that smokers using the 'will-power' method make is waiting to become a non-smoker. They are waiting for nothing to happen. When you come out of the dentist, your jaw might still be aching, but are you miserable? Of course not. You are delighted that the visit is over and don't sit waiting for the pain to go.

It is only the waiting and doubting that create the problem. If you watch the milk boil, it won't. Take your eye off it for a micro-second and it will be all over the stove. You don't sit and watch paint dry. What is the point of waiting not to smoke any more?

Get it clearly into your mind: you aren't giving up living. You aren't giving up anything. In fact, you are going to enjoy social occasions more and be better equipped to handle stress the moment you cut off the supply of nicotine. The only thing that can prevent you from succeeding is doubt and uncertainty.

You know you've made the correct decision, so for the next few days and for the rest of your life never, ever question that decision. Get it into your mind that there is no such thing as one cigarette, or an occasional cigarette, or special cigarettes. It's that one cigarette that gets us hooked in the first place and it's just one cigarette that gets us into the trap again. It's also the thoughts of occasional cigarettes or special cigarettes that keep smokers who quit by using the 'will-power' method vulnerable for the rest of their lives.

The real difference between a smoker and a non-smoker is that non-smokers have no need or desire to smoke a single cigarette. If you continue to see one cigarette as some sort of crutch or pleasure, you'll see a million cigarettes as some sort of crutch or pleasure. The only choice you'll have will be to be like the complaining stoppers and spend the rest of your life feeling deprived and miserable because you aren't allowed to have one, or you'll succumb, get hooked again and be even more miserable.

Why torture yourself? Accept for the next few days the fact that the little monster might trigger the thought: "I want a cigarette." When I tried the 'will-power' method it would happen every morning. I'd wake up and think: "I'll get up and have a cigarette." Then I'd remember that I'd 'given up'. It was like black depression. I'd think: "I'm not allowed to smoke any more, who wants to give up?" When you extinguish that final cigarette, look forward to spending the rest of the day without a cigarette, so proving to yourself that you can both cope with life and enjoy life without them. As you lie in bed that night, prepare yourself for the next day. Don't think: "How will I survive a whole day without a cigarette?"

Look forward to the exciting challenge of proving that you can cope with life and enjoy life for a whole day.

I must make it clear – lest you confuse my advice with A.A.'s dictum of 'Take each day as it comes', or the attitude of a 'will-power' stopper, "I've survived 3 days 4 hours and 22 minutes." No, those are depressive attitudes, waiting and hoping that the misery will end. Rather see it in the same light as a lottery winner who is looking forward to tomorrow with excitement.

Another mistake of the 'will-power' stoppers is to avoid social situations where they feel they might be tempted. No wonder they feel so miserable. Remember, you haven't given up living, you haven't given up anything. Go straight away to parties and meals. If there are 20 smokers there and just you, remember that every one of those smokers would love to be like you.

Often on such occasions you forget you have quit. The cigarettes are being handed around and you suddenly find yourself reaching for one. Your 'friend' says: "I thought you'd quit." You feel stupid, hand stuck in the air. It's at times like this that doubt creeps in and you start to question your decision. Don't, this is just the time to reinforce it. Just a few months ago I went to look out of my car window. I went to take the cigarette out of my mouth before I did so. I felt stupid; there was no cigarette there. Had I stopped with the 'will-power' method, this incident would have hurt me deeply. My attitude would have been: "I haven't smoked for over 14 years but I still haven't broken the habit. Instead it was the complete opposite: 14 years ago that cigarette would have been stuck in my mouth, my teeth and upper lip would have been nicotine stained, the ashtray would have been overflowing with butts and the roof of the car would have been yellow or brown. Thank God, I'm free.

Perhaps you are under the impression that you will have to abstain 14 years for that to happen to you. No, that was my attitude even before I'd extinguished the final cigarette. Perhaps you think it was a form of positive thinking, a device to make me believe I didn't need to smoke. No, I've always been a positive thinker. I can't kid myself. When I believed I needed to smoke, I had to smoke, even though I knew it was killing me. Once I saw through the confidence trick there was no way I could have continued to smoke even if I'd wanted to kid myself.

If it happens to you at a party, be prepared, but don't worry about it. Just say to the smokers: "I'd forgotten I had quit and I can't tell you how lovely it is to be free. You should try it." Since smoking became anti-social and so many smokers have managed to quit, every smoker is terrified that they'll be the last to leave the sinking ship, or, even worse, that they'll go down with it. Even if it is someone that loves you, one part of them will hate you because you have managed to escape from the sinking ship and have left them feeling even more isolated.

They'll hate you even more because they'll expect you to be miserable and depressed, whereas you actually enjoy being a non-smoker. Let me refer you back to the dinner party, and in particular to the girl that had quit for eight years but was still craving a cigarette. Can you imagine the effect that had on the other girl who was probably convinced that she couldn't quit for a day let alone eight years!

It is these complaining stoppers who convince the rest of us that we can never be free. Although one part of your friend's brain will hate you, you will actually help her. You will not only shortly experience your own joy of being free, but the additional joy of helping others to be free. This is the wonderful thing that is happening today. Millions of smokers have managed to escape, and when your friend sees that you are not only free but actually enjoying the process, you will help to remove his or her fear of quitting.

For the next few days you will be achieving something wonderful, enjoy being the focus of attention. Your family, work colleagues and friends will expect you to whinge and be miserable. When they see you happy and enjoying life they will think you are Superman or Superwoman. The important thing is that you will be feeling like Superman or Superwoman.

It's other smokers that get us hooked in the first place and it is other smokers that make us feel we are missing out if we do manage to quit. If you should ever feel deprived in the company of a smoker, remember that when they leave your company they have to continue to smoke. The next cancer scare, the next time their lungs are congested, the next time their loved ones give them that frightened look, the next time they are not allowed to smoke, the next time they feel stupid or unclean because they are the lone smoker in the company of non-smokers, they have to go on smoking, and what pleasure or crutch do they get in return?

ABSOLUTELY NONE

Just think of this as a piece of market research. Not only is every non-smoker in the world happy to be a non-smoker, but every smoker in the world wishes they had never become hooked. That's pretty conclusive!

Also remember, that whenever you see a smoker light up, whether it be a cigarette, cigar or pipe, whether it be a stressful, social or boring situation, they are not doing so because they choose to. If you ever find yourself envying a smoker, remember that it is they that are being deprived and not you. They are being deprived of their health, their energy, their money, their self-respect, their courage, their confidence, their freedom:

THEY ARE DRUG ADDICTS

You wouldn't envy a heroin addict. In the UK, heroin kills fewer than 100 addicts yearly; smoking kills 2,000 every week and over 3,500,000 smokers worldwide every year. Like all drug addiction, it doesn't get better; it's like sinking gradually and imperceptibly into a bottomless pit. If you don't like being a smoker today, no way will you enjoy being one tomorrow.

Now rejoice in the fact that you can now smoke:

THE FINAL CIGARETTE

31

THE FINAL CIGARETTE

If you have understood everything that I have said, by now you should be impatient to get going. If so, you are free to go. Perhaps you feel that you have understood everything that I have said but are still apprehensive. It might just be fear of failure. If so, don't worry; just as a ladder will get you to the top of a wall, provided it's long enough and provided you use it properly, so Easyway will enable any smoker to find it easy to quit, providing they follow all the instructions.

The key is to be certain. If you find that you cannot believe everything that I have said, then you need to re-read or consult one of our clinics. If you have understood but are still apprehensive, don't worry; some people find that the proof of the pudding is in the eating. Provided you follow all the instructions, and, in particular, the instruction of starting off in a happy frame of mind, you will find that after just a few days you will have a moment, it might be a stressful situation, a social situation, whatever – one of those situations that you thought you could never cope with or enjoy without a cigarette. It suddenly occurs to you, that not only did you cope with it, or enjoy it, it never even occurred to you to light a cigarette. That is The Moment of Revelation, the moment that you realize that you are free. However, if you wait for it or try to make it happen, you create a phobia – it's the same as trying not to think about it. The whole key is to extinguish that final cigarette with a feeling of relief and excitement, and get on with enjoying the rest of your life.

Some smokers are like me and can see the confidence trick so clearly that they receive The Moment of Revelation even before they have smoked the final cigarette. Often such smokers will ask me: "Do I really need to smoke the final cigarette? You've explained it so clearly, I know I will never be tempted to smoke again."

It seems silly that someone like me, who loathes smoking so much, should advise someone to smoke one final cigarette. I do so only because I know how essential it is to know how important it is to be certain. I need you now to make a solemn vow that when you extinguish this last cigarette:

YOU WILL NEVER EVER SMOKE ANOTHER

I need you to make a further vow, that from this day forth, whenever you think about smoking, whether it be a good day or a bad day, you never question your decision, but simply think:

YIPPEE! I'M A NON-SMOKER!

I never tire of reading the comments of other smokers who have escaped from the nicotine prison. I would love to hear your comments, critical or otherwise. Write to me care of one of my clinics; a list of these is provided in the back of the book.

I won't wish you luck. You don't need it. Just follow the instructions. (These are listed in brief in the next section for easy reference.)

Best wishes.

INSTRUCTIONS

A: WHILE READING THE BOOK

• FOLLOW ALL THE INSTRUCTIONS TO THE LETTER

• START OFF WITH A FEELING OF ELATION

• CONTINUE TO SMOKE WHILE READING THE BOOK

• KEEP AN OPEN MIND

B: PRIOR TO AND AFTER THE RITUAL OF THE FINAL CIGARETTE

• EXTINGUISH THAT CIGARETTE WITH A FEELING OF FREEDOM AND ELATION – NOT DEPRIVATION.

• BE AWARE THAT THE LITTLE MONSTER WILL BE TRYING TO TRICK YOU. IF YOU GET THE FEELING OF "I WANT A CIGARETTE", REMEMBER IT'S JUST HIS DEATH THROES. REJOICE IN THEM.

• REMEMBER SMOKING DOES ABSOLUTELY NOTHING FOR YOU. ON THE CONTRARY, IT IS JUST AN ILLUSION. IT DOES THE COMPLETE OPPOSITE.

• DO NOT AVOID SMOKERS OR SMOKING SITUATIONS OR CHANGE YOUR LIFESTYLE IN ANY WAY BECAUSE YOU HAVE QUIT SMOKING. REMEMBER, YOU ARE GIVING UP NOTHING. ON THE CONTRARY, YOU ARE FREEING YOURSELF OF A TERRIBLE DISEASE.

• DO NOT ENVY OTHER SMOKERS. REMEMBER, EVERY ONE OF THEM WOULD LOVE TO BE FREE LIKE YOU!

• REMEMBER, THERE IS NO SUCH THING AS JUST ONE CIGARETTE. SMOKING IS NICOTINE ADDICTION AND A LIFETIME'S CHAIN OF MISERY.

• DO NOT WAIT TO BECOME A NON-SMOKER. YOU BECAME A NON-SMOKER THE MOMENT YOU CUT OFF THE SUPPLY OF NICOTINE!

• DO NOT TRY NOT TO THINK ABOUT SMOKING AND DO NOT WORRY IF YOUR THOUGHTS ARE OBSESSED BY SMOKING FOR A FEW DAYS. BUT WHENEVER YOU DO THINK ABOUT IT, NEVER EVER QUESTION YOUR DECISION. YOU KNOW IT'S CORRECT. JUST GET INTO THE HABIT OF THINKING:

YIPPEE! I'M A NON-SMOKER!

ALLEN CARR'S EASYWAY CLINICS

The following pages list contact details for all Allen Carr Stop Smoking Clinics worldwide where the success rate, based on the money back guarantee, is over 90%.
Selected clinics also offer sessions that deal with alcohol and weight issues. Please check with your nearest clinic, which is listed, for details.
Allen Carr guarantees you will find it easy to stop smoking at his clinics or your money back.

Worldwide Head Office
Park House, 14 Pepys Road,
Raynes Park, London SW20 8NH
Tel: +44 (0)20 8944 7761
Email: mail@allencarr.com
Website: www.allencarr.com
Worldwide Press Office
Tel: +44 (0)7970 88 44 52
Email: jd@statacom.net

UK Clinic Information and Central Booking Line
Tel: 0800 389 2115 (Freephone)

UK CLINICS

London
Park House, 14 Pepys Road,
Raynes Park, SW20 8NH
Tel: +44 (0)20 8944 7761
Fax: +44 (0)20 8944 8619
Therapists: John Dicey, Colleen Dwyer, Crispin Hay, Emma Sole, Rob Fielding, James Pyper
Email: mail@allencarr.com

Aylesbury
Tel: 0800 0197 017
Therapists: Kim Bennett,
Emma Sole
Email: kim@easywaybucks.co.uk

Belfast
Tel: 0845 094 3244
Therapist: Tara Evers-Cheung
Email: tara@easywayni.com

Birmingham
415 Hagley Road West, Quinton, B32 2AD
Tel & Fax: +44 (0)121 423 1227
Therapists: John Dicey, Colleen Dwyer, Crispin Hay, Rob Fielding

Email: easywayadmin@
btconnect.com

Bournemouth
Tel: 0800 028 7257 / +44 (0)1425 272 757
Therapists: John Dicey, Colleen Dwyer, Emma Sole, James Pyper
Email: easywayadmin@
btconnect.com

Brighton
Tel: 0800 028 7257
Therapists: John Dicey, Colleen Dwyer, Emma Sole, James Pyper
Email: easywayadmin@
btconnect.com

Bristol
Tel: +44 (0)117 950 1441
Therapist: Charles Holdsworth Hunt
Email: stopsmoking@
easywaybristol.co.uk

Cambridge
Tel: 0800 0197 017
Therapists: Kim Bennett,
Emma Sole
Email: kim@easywaybucks.co.uk

Cardiff
Tel: +44 (0)117 950 1441
Therapist: Charles Holdsworth Hunt
E-mail: stopsmoking@
easywaybristol.co.uk

Coventry
Tel: 0800 321 3007
Therapist: Rob Fielding
Email: info@easywaycoventry.co.uk

Crewe
Tel: +44 (0)1270 501 487
Therapist: Debbie Brewer-West
Email: debbie@
easyway2stopsmoking.co.uk

Cumbria
Tel: 0800 077 6187
Therapist: Mark Keen
Email: mark@
easywaycumbria.co.uk

Derby
Tel: 0800 0197 017
Therapists: Kim Bennett,
Emma Sole
Email: kim@easywaybucks.co.uk

Essex
Tel: 0800 389 2115

Exeter
Tel: +44 (0)117 950 1441
Therapist: Charles
Holdsworth Hunt
Email: stopsmoking@
easywayexeter.co.uk

High Wycombe
Tel: 0800 0197 017
Therapists: Kim Bennett,
Emma Sole
Email: kim@easywaybucks.co.uk

Ipswich
Website: www.allencarr.com

Kent
Tel: 0800 028 7257
Therapists: John Dicey, Colleen Dwyer, Emma
Sole, James Pyper
Lancashire
Tel: 0800 077 6187
Therapist: Mark Keen
Email: mark@
easywaylancashire.co.uk

Leeds
Tel: 0800 804 6796
Therapist: Rob Groves
Email: stopsmoking@
easywayyorkshire.co.uk

Leicester
Tel: 0800 321 3007
Therapist: Rob Fielding
Email: info@easywayleicester.co.uk

Lincoln
Tel: 0800 321 3007
Therapist: Rob Fielding

Liverpool
Tel: 0800 077 6187
Therapist: Mark Keen
Email: mark@
easywayliverpool.co.uk

Manchester
Freephone: 0800 804 6796
Therapist: Rob Groves
Email: stopsmoking@
easywaymanchester.co.uk

Milton Keynes
Tel: 0800 0197 017
Therapists: Kim Bennett,
Emma Sole
Email: kim@easywaybucks.co.uk
Newcastle/North East
Tel & Fax: +44 (0)191 581 0449
Therapist: Tony Attrill
Email: info@stopsmoking-uk.net

Northampton
Tel: 0800 0197 017
Therapists: Kim Bennett,
Emma Sole
Email: kim@easywaybucks.co.uk

Norwich
Website: www.allencarr.com

Nottingham
Tel: 0800 0197 017
Therapists: Kim Bennett,
Emma Sole
Email: kim@easywaybucks.co.uk

Oxford
Tel: 0800 0197 017
Therapists: Kim Bennett,
Emma Sole
Email: kim@easywaybucks.co.uk

Peterborough
Tel: 0800 0197 017
Therapists: Kim Bennett,
Emma Sole
Email: kim@easywaybucks.co.uk

Reading
Tel: 0800 028 7257
Therapists: John Dicey, Colleen Dwyer, Emma
Sole, James Pyper

SCOTLAND
Glasgow and Edinburgh
Tel: +44 (0)131 449 7858
Therapists: Paul Melvin and
Jim McCreadie
Email: info@easywayscotland.co.uk

Sheffield
Tel: 0800 804 6796
Therapist: Rob Groves
Email: stopsmoking@
easywayyorkshire.co.uk

Shrewsbury
Tel: +44 (0)1270 501 487
Therapist: Debbie Brewer-West
Email: debbie@
easyway2stopsmoking.co.uk

Southampton
Tel: 0800 028 7257 / +44 (0)1425 272 757
Therapists: John Dicey, Colleen Dwyer, Emma
Sole, James Pyper
Email: easywayadmin@tiscali.co.uk

Southport
Tel: 0800 077 6187
Therapist: Mark Keen
Email: mark@
easywaylancashire.co.uk

Staines/Heathrow
Tel: 0800 028 7257
Therapists: John Dicey, Colleen Dwyer, Emma
Sole, James Pyper

Surrey
Park House, 14 Pepys Road, Raynes Park,
London SW20 8NH
Tel: +44 (0)20 8944 7761
Fax: +44 (0)20 8944 8619
Therapists: John Dicey, Colleen Dwyer, Crispin
Hay, Emma Sole, Rob Fielding, James Pyper

Email: mail@allencarr.com

Stevenage
Tel: 0800 019 7017
Therapists: Kim Bennett,
Emma Sole
Email: kim@easywaybucks.co.uk

Stoke
Tel: +44 (0)1270 501 487
Therapist: Debbie Brewer-West
Email: debbie@
easyway2stopsmoking.co.uk

Swindon
Tel: +44 (0)117 950 1441
Therapist: Charles
Holdsworth Hunt
Email: stopsmoking@
easywaybristol.co.uk

Telford
Tel: +44 (0)1270 501487
Therapist: Debbie Brewer-West
Email: debbie@
easyway2stopsmoking.co.uk

Worcester
Tel: 0800 321 3007
Therapist: Rob Fielding

WORLDWIDE CLINICS

REPUBLIC OF IRELAND
Dublin and Cork
Lo-Call (From ROI) 1 890 ESYWAY (37 99 29)
Tel: +353 (0)1 499 9010 (4 lines)
Therapists: Brenda Sweeney
and Team
Email: info@allencarr.ie

AUSTRALIA
North Queensland
Tel: 1300 85 11 75
Therapist: Tara Pickard-Clark
Email: nqld@allencarr.com.au

Sydney, New South Wales
Tel & Fax: 1300 78 51 80
Therapist: Natalie Clays
Email: nsw@allencarr.com.au

South Australia
Therapist: Phillip Collins
Freecall: 1300 88 60 31
Email: sa@allencarr.com.au

South Queensland
Tel: 1300 85 58 06
Therapist: Jonathan Wills
Email: sqld@allencarr.com.au

Victoria, Tasmania, Act.
Tel: +61 (0)3 9894 8866
or 1300 790 565 (Freecall)
Therapist: Gail Morris
Email: info@allencarr.com.au
Western Australia
Therapist: Dianne Fisher
Tel: 1300 55 78 01
Email: wa@allencarr.com.au

AUSTRIA
(Sessions held throughout Austria)
Free line telephone for Information
and Booking:
0800RAUCHEN (0800 7282436)
Triesterstraße 42, 8724 Spielberg
Tel: +43 (0)3512 44755
Therapists: Erich Kellermann
and Team
Email: info@allen-carr.at

BELGIUM
Antwerp
Koningin Astridplein 27 B-9150 Bazel
Tel: +32 (0)3 281 6255
Fax: +32 (0)3 744 0608
Therapist: Dirk Nielandt
Email: easyway@dirknielandt.be

BULGARIA
Tel: 0800 14104
Therapist: Rumyana Kostadinova
Email: rumyana.kostadinova@
easyway.bg

CANADA
Toll free: +1-866 666 4299 / +1 905 849 7736
Therapist: Damian O'Hara
Seminars held in Toronto
and Vancouver
Corporate programs available throughout
Canada
Email: info@
theeasywaytostopsmoking.com

CHILE
Tel: +56 2 4744587
Therapist: Claudia Sarmiento
Email: contacto@allencarr.cl

COLOMBIA
Bogota
Tel: +57 1 245 6910
Therapist: Jose Manuel Duran
Email: easywaycolombia@
cable.net.co

CYPRUS
Tel: +357 77 77 78 30
Therapist: Kyriacos Michaelides
Email: info@allencarr.com.cy

CZECH REPUBLIC
Tel: +42 (0) 257 325 117
Therapist: Adriana Gasparova
Email: office@allencarr.cz

DENMARK
Sessions held throughout Denmark
Tel: +45 70267711
Therapist: Mette Fonss
Email: mette@easyway.dk

ECUADOR
Tel & Fax: +593 (0)2 2820 920
Therapist: Ingrid Wittich
Email: toisan@pi.pro.ec

ESTONIA – opening 2009
Website: www.allencarr.com

FRANCE
Sessions held throughout France
Central Booking Line: 0800 FUMEUR
(Freephone)
Therapists: Erick Serre and Team
Tel: +33 (4) 91 33 54 55
Email: info@allencarr.fr

GERMANY
Sessions held throughout Germany
Free line telephone for information and central
booking line: 08000RAUCHEN (0800
07282436)
Therapists: Erich Kellermann
and Team
Kirchenweg 41, D-83026 Rosenheim
Tel: +49 (0) 8031 90190-0
Email: info@allen-carr.de

GREECE
Sessions held throughout Greece
Tel: +30 210 5224087
Therapist: Panos Tzouras
Email: panos@allencarr.gr

ICELAND
Reykjavik
Tel: +354 553 9590
Therapist: Petur Einarsson
Email: easyway@easyway.is

INDIA
Bangalore & Chennai
Tel: +91 (0)80 41540624
Therapist: Suresh Shottam
Email: info@
easywaytostopsmoking.co.in

ISRAEL
Sessions held throughout Israel
Tel: +972 (0)3 6212525
Therapists: Ramy Romanovsky, Orit Rozen,
Shahaf Ashkenazi, Kinneret Triffon
Email: info@allencarr.co.il

ITALY
Sessions held throughout Italy
Tel/Fax: +39 (0)2 7060 2438
Therapists: Francesca Cesati
and Team
Email: info@easywayitalia.com

JAPAN
Sessions held throughout Japan
Tel: +81 3 5288 5177
Therapist: Miho Shimada
Email: info@allen-carr.jp

LATVIA – opening 2009
Website: www.allencarr.com

LITHUANIA
Tel: +370 694 29591
Therapist: Evaldas Zvirblis
Email: info@mestirukyti.eu
Website: www.allencarr.com

MAURITIUS
Tel: +230 727 5103
Therapist: Heidi Houreau
Email: allencarrmauritius@
yahoo.com

MEXICO
Sessions held throughout Mexico
Tel: +52 55 2623 0631
Therapists: Jorge Davo and Mario Campuzano
Otero
Email: info@allencarr-mexico.com

NETHERLANDS
Amsterdam
Tel: +31 (0)20 465 4665 Fax: +31 (0)20 465
6682
Therapist: Eveline de Mooij
Email: amsterdam@allencarr.nl

Utrecht
Tel: +31 (0)35 602 94 58
Therapist: Paula Rooduijn
Email: soest@allencarr.nl

Rotterdam
Tel: +31 (0)10 244 0709
Fax: +31 (0)10 244 07 10
Therapist: Kitty van't Hof
Email: rotterdam@allencarr.nl

Nijmegen
Tel: +31 (0)24 360 33 05
Therapist: Jacqueline van den Bosch
Email: nijmegen@allencarr.nl

NEW ZEALAND
North Island – Auckland
Tel: +64 (0)9 817 5396
Therapist: Vickie Macrae
Email: vickie@easywaynz.co.nz

South Island – Christchurch
Tel: +64 (0)3 326 5464
Therapist: Laurence Cooke
Email: laurence@
easywaysouthisland.co.nz

NORWAY
Oslo
Tel: +47 93 20 09 11
Therapist: René Adde
Email: post@easyway-norge.no

POLAND
Sessions held throughout Poland
Tel: +48 (0)22 621 36 11
Therapist: Anna Kabat
Email: info@allen-carr.pl

PORTUGAL
Oporto
Tel: +351 22 9958698
Therapist: Ria Slof
Email: info@
comodeixardefumar.com

MOSCOW – opening 2009
Website: www.allencarr.com

SERBIA
Belgrade
Tel: +381 (0)11 308 8686
Email: milos.rakovic@
allencarrserbia.com/
office@allencarr.co.yu

SINGAPORE
Tel: +65 6329 9660
Therapist: Pam Oei
Email: pam@allencarr.com.sg

SLOVAKIA
Tel: +421 55 678 26 55
Therapist: Adriana Gasparova
Email: office@allencarr.sk

SLOVENIA – opening 2009
Website:www.allencarr.com

SOUTH AFRICA
Sessions held throughout South Africa
Central Booking Line: 0861 100 200
Head Office
15 Draper Square, Draper St, Claremont 7708
Cape Town
Tel: +27 (0)21 851 5883
Mobile: 083 600 5555
Therapists: Dr Charles Nel,
Dudley Garner, Malcolm Robinson and Team
Email: easyway@allencarr.co.za

SPAIN
Website: www.allencarr.com

SWEDEN
Goteborge & Malmö
Tel: +46 (0)31 24 01 00
Email: info@allencarr.nu

Stockholm
Tel: +46 (0)8 743 09 50
Therapist: Christofer Elde
Email: info@allencarr.se

SWITZERLAND
Sessions held throughout Switzerland
Freephone for Information and Booking:
0800RAUCHEN (0800/728 2436)
Tel: +41 (0)52 383 3773
Fax: +41 (0)52 3833774
Therapists: Cyrill Argast and Team
For sessions in Suisse Romand; and Svizzera
Italiana:
Tel: 0800 386 387
Email: info@allen-carr.ch

TURKEY
Sessions held throughout Turkey
Tel: +90 212 358 5307
Therapist: Emre Ustunucar
Email: info@allencarrturkiye.com

USA
Sessions held throughout the USA
Central information and bookings
(Toll Free): 1 866 666 4299
Email: info@
theeasywaytostopsmoking.com
Seminars held regularly in New York,
Los Angeles, Denver and Houston
Corporate programs available throughout
the USA
Mailing address: 1133 Broadway, Suite 706, New
York, NY 10010
Therapists: Damian O'Hara, Collene Curran

DISCOUNT VOUCHER
for
ALLEN CARR'S
EASYWAY CLINICS

Recover the price of this book when you attend an
Allen Carr's Easyway to Stop Smoking
Clinic anywhere in the world!

Allen Carr has a global network of clinics where
he guarantees you will find it easy to stop
smoking or your money back.

**The success rate based on this
money back guarantee is over 90%.**

When you book your session mention this
voucher and you will receive a discount to
the value of this book. Contact your nearest
clinic for more information on how the sessions
work and to book your appointment.

**Details of Allen Carr's Easyway
Clinics can be found at**
www.allencarr.com
or call **0800 389 2115**

Easyway To Stop Drinking Alcohol
sessions are available at limited locations.
Call +44 (0)20 8944 7761 for latest listings.